Navigating Life
with Epilepsy

Lisa M. Shulman, MD

Editor-in-Chief, *Neurology Now*™ Books Series
Fellow of the American Academy of Neurology
Professor of Neurology
The Eugenia Brin Professor in Parkinson's Disease and Movement Disorders
The Rosalyn Newman Distinguished Scholar in Parkinson's Disease
Director, University of Maryland PD & Movement Disorders Center
University of Maryland School of Medicine
Baltimore, MD

Other Titles in the *Neurology Now*™ Books Series

Navigating Life with Parkinson's Disease
Sortirios A. Parashos, MD, PhD; Rose Wichmann, PT; and Todd Melby

Navigating Life with a Brain Tumor
Lynne P. Taylor, MD, FAAN; Alyx B. Porter Umphrey, MD; and Diane Richard

Navigating the Complexities of Stroke
Louis R. Caplan, MD, FAAN

Navigating Life with Multiple Sclerosis
Kathleen Costello, MS, ANP-BC, MSCN; Ben W. Thrower, MD;
and Barbara S. Giesser, MD

Navigating Life

with Epilepsy

David C. Spencer, MD, FAAN

Professor of Neurology
Director, Oregon Health & Science University Epilepsy Program
Portland, Oregon

AMERICAN ACADEMY OF
NEUROLOGY.

OXFORD
UNIVERSITY PRESS

OXFORD
UNIVERSITY PRESS

Oxford University Press is a department of the University of Oxford. It furthers
the University's objective of excellence in research, scholarship, and education
by publishing worldwide. Oxford is a registered trade mark of Oxford University
Press in the UK and certain other countries.

Published in the United States of America by Oxford University Press
198 Madison Avenue, New York, NY 10016, United States of America.

Library of Congress Cataloging-in-Publication Data is available on request.
ISBN 978–0–19–935895–3

3 5 7 9 8 6 4
Printed by Sheridan Books, Inc., United States of America

CONTENTS

ABOUT THE AAN'S *NEUROLOGY NOW*™ BOOKS SERIES

Here is a question for you:

If you know more about your neurologic condition, will you do better than if you know less?

Well, not simply optimism but hard data show that individuals who are more knowledgeable about their medical conditions *do have better outcomes*. So learning about your neurologic condition plays an important role in doing the very best you can. The main purpose of both the *Neurology Now*™ Books series and *Neurology Now* magazine from American Academy of Neurology (AAN) and American Brain Foundation (ABF) is to focus on the needs of people with neurologic disorders. Our goal is to view neurologic issues through the eyes of people with neurologic problems, in order to understand and respond to their practical day-to-day needs.

So, you are probably saying, *"Of course, knowledge is a good thing, but how can it change the course of my disease?"* Well, health care is really a two-way street. After you have had a stroke, you need to find a knowledgeable and trusted neurologist; however, no physician can overcome the obstacle of working with inaccurate or incomplete information. Your physician is working to navigate the clues you provide in your own words combined with the clues from their neurologic examination, in order to arrive at an accurate diagnosis and respond to your individual needs. Many types of important clues exist, such as your description of your symptoms or your ability to identify how your neurologic condition affects your daily activities. Poor patient–physician communication inevitably results in less-than-ideal outcomes. This problem is well described by the old adage, "garbage in, garbage out." The better you pin down and communicate your main problem(s), the more likely you are to walk out of your doctor's office with the plan that is right for you. Your neurologist is the expert in your disorder, but you and your family are the experts in "you." Physician decision making is not a "one shoe fits all" enterprise, yet when accurate, individualized information is lacking, that's what it becomes.

Whether you are startled by hearing a new diagnosis or you come to this knowledge gradually, learning that you have a neurologic problem is jarring. Many neurologic disorders are chronic; you aren't simply adjusting to something new—you will need to deal with this disorder for the foreseeable future. In certain ways, life has changed. Now, there are two crucial "next steps": the first is finding good neurologic care for your problem, and the second is successfully adjusting to living with your condition. This second step depends on attaining knowledge of your condition, learning new skills to manage the condition, and finding the flexibility and resourcefulness to restore your quality of life. When successful, you regain your equilibrium and restore a sense of confidence and control that is the cornerstone of well-being.

When healthy adjustment does not occur following a new diagnosis, a sense of feeling out of control and overwhelmed often persists, and no doctor's prescription will adequately respond to this problem. Individuals who acquire good self-management skills are often able to recognize and understand new symptoms and take appropriate action. Conversely, those who are lacking in confidence may respond to the same symptom with a growing sense of anxiety and urgency. In the first case, "watchful waiting" or a call to the physician may result in resolution of the problem. In the second case, the uncertainty and anxiety often lead to multiple physician consultations, unnecessary new prescriptions, social withdrawal, or unwarranted hospitalization. Outcomes can be dramatically different depending on knowledge and preparedness.

Managing a neurologic disorder is new territory, and you should not be surprised that you need to be equipped with new information and a new skill set to effectively manage your condition. You will need to learn new words that describe both your symptoms and their treatment to communicate effectively with the members of your medical team. You will also need to learn how to gather accurate information about your condition when you need it and to avoid misinformation. Although all of your physicians document your progress in their medical records, keeping a personal journal about your neurologic condition will help you summarize and track all your medical information in one place. When you bring this journal with you as you go to see your physician, you will be able to provide more accurate information about your history and previous treatment. Your active and informed involvement in your care and decision making results in a better quality of care and better outcomes.

Your neurologic condition is likely to pose new challenges in daily activities, including interactions in your family, your workplace, and your social and recreational activities. How can you best manage your symptoms or your medication dosing schedule in the context of your normal activities? When should you disclose your diagnosis to others? *Neurology Now* Books provide you with the background you need, including the experiences of others who have faced similar problems, to guide you through this unfamiliar terrain. Our goal is to give you the resources you need to "take your doctor with you" when you confront these new challenges. We are committed to answering the questions and concerns of individuals living with neurologic disorders and their families in each volume of the *Neurology Now* Books series. We want you to be as prepared and confident as possible to participate with your doctors in your medical care. Much care is taken to develop each book with you in mind. We include the most up-to-date, informative, and useful answers to the questions that most concern you—whether you find yourself in the unexpected role of patient or caregiver. Real-life experiences of patients and families are found throughout the text to illustrate important points. And feedback based on correspondence from *Neurology Now* magazine readers informs topics for new books and is integral to our quality improvement. These features are found in all books in the *Neurology Now* Books series so that you can expect the same quality and patient-centered approach in every volume.

I hope that you have arrived at a new understanding of why "knowledge is empowering" when it comes to your medical care and that *Neurology Now* Books will serve as an important foundation for the new skills you need to be effective in managing a neurologic condition.

Lisa M. Shulman, MD
Editor-in-Chief, *Neurology Now*™ Books Series
Fellow of the American Academy of Neurology
Professor of Neurology
The Eugenia Brin Professor in Parkinson's Disease
and Movement Disorders
The Rosalyn Newman Distinguished Scholar
in Parkinson's Disease
Director, University of Maryland PD &
Movement Disorders Center
University of Maryland School of Medicine

ACKNOWLEDGMENTS

I am grateful to Sara Taggart, W. Brewster Smith, MD, Lisa Shulman, MD, and Andrea Weiss for their review and helpful comments, to the editorial team at Oxford University Press, to my family for their support, and finally to my patients, who have taught me what it means to have epilepsy.

Navigating Life
with Epilepsy

Chapter 1

Introduction

Sebastian didn't used to think about having a seizure when he left the house. In fact, he took his good health for granted. Shortly after he turned 17, he had his first seizure. He had just gotten out of school for the summer, and had stayed up late with his friends the night before. His family was planning to spend the weekend at the beach, and he got up early to help load the car. The next thing he remembered, he was in the emergency department and people were asking him what day it was and who was the president. He had a headache, his whole body ached, and his tongue was sore. He soon learned that his family had witnessed his first **generalized tonic-clonic** (GTC, sometimes referred to as "**grand mal**") seizure.

Three months and three seizures later, a lot of things were different for Sebastian. Everyone was worried about him, although his parents were starting to hover over him a little less. He couldn't drive. He had to see a new doctor—a neurologist—who put him through a bunch of tests and started him on medication. Everything seemed to be happening so fast, and he still had a lot of questions about what was going on. Why did he start having seizures? When would he be able to drive? What did his friends and schoolmates think? How long would he have to stay on this medication? Sebastian was beginning to experience what it means to live with epilepsy.

Like Sebastian, maybe you, a friend, or a family member has been diagnosed recently with epilepsy. Or maybe epilepsy has been part of your life for years. Whether epilepsy is new or familiar, this book will have something for you.

Literally millions of people before Sebastian have had similar questions and concerns. One study asked people with epilepsy to list their top concerns related to the condition. The most frequently reported concern was about driving. This was followed by concerns about independence, work, social embarrassment, medication dependence, mood and stress, and safety.

The concerns of each individual are unique, but there are many common threads. This book strives to provide answers for your questions and reassurance that your concerns have been successfully navigated by many others before you. It focuses on issues in adolescents and adults with epilepsy. Because it is not unusual for certain forms of epilepsy to begin in childhood and then persist into adolescence and adulthood, some reference will be made to childhood epilepsy. However, this book is not a guide to managing epilepsy in children. If your main interest is in learning about seizures and epilepsy in infants and children, there are several excellent options for more reading (see **Appendix 1**).

In simplest terms, epilepsy is a condition marked by recurrent, unprovoked seizures. It is exceedingly common—nearly 1 percent of the population in developed countries has epilepsy—and the rate is even higher in the developing world. Epilepsy can appear at any age, but most commonly begins either in childhood or after the age of 65. It affects men and women equally, and is common in people of all ethnic groups. I am a neurologist and epilepsy specialist who has been providing care and education for people with epilepsy for nearly two decades. When I give lectures about epilepsy, I often begin by having audience members raise a hand if they have a friend or family member with epilepsy. Often more than half of the audience has a hand raised.

Historical Roots and Stigma

This brings up a paradox about epilepsy. It is very common, so many people are familiar with it and have friends and family members with seizures. Yet too often, there is still a negative or shameful value attached to epilepsy, and the stigma attached to the condition remains. This stigma can take many forms, from subtle social discrimination, to job discrimination, to complete social isolation in some cultures. Important strides have been made, including a World Health Organization campaign in the late 1990s to bring epilepsy "Out of the Shadows." Education plays a major role in eliminating stigma, as it often arises from ignorance and fear. It is my hope that this book will help minimize the stigma that you and your family may experience.

Some of this stigma grows from the historical roots of epilepsy. Descriptions of epilepsy were first recorded thousands of years ago, including as far back as 1000 B.C. in ancient Babylonia. In these ancient texts, seizures and epilepsy were often well described. However, it was not understood that epilepsy was a brain disease. Instead, it was thought of as a spiritual disorder. Despite improved understanding of epilepsy by the ancient Greeks, including Hippocrates, this misunderstanding of epilepsy as an affliction by evil spirits persisted for many years. Although seizures were sometimes viewed as a sign of divine inspiration, more commonly they were viewed as the work of evil spirits or demonic possession. Gross misunderstanding of the condition and inadequate treatments persisted through the middle ages. It was not until the eighteenth and nineteenth centuries that the concept of epilepsy as a brain disease was firmly established and expanded upon. By the end of the nineteenth century, the first moderately effective treatment for epilepsy (potassium bromide) was developed and widely used.

Woven through this historical fabric are stories of famous men and women with epilepsy. Limitations of the historical record and medical diagnosis at the time make it difficult to firmly establish the diagnosis of epilepsy in some cases. However, many prominent historical figures and great thinkers were believed to have had epilepsy, including Socrates, Aristotle, Julius Caesar, Peter the Great, and Napoleon. Many famous writers and artists throughout history appear on the list, including Charles Dickens, Fyodor Dostoyevsky, and Vincent van Gogh. Modern-day celebrities with epilepsy include actor Danny Glover, musicians Prince and Neil Young, and doubtless numerous others who have not chosen to share their condition with the public.

Many famous sports figures have epilepsy, and several have become advocates for people with epilepsy. One of the many such compelling figures from the world of sports is Chanda Gunn. Chanda had her first seizures and diagnosis of epilepsy at age 9. An avid swimmer, she was told that she should not surf or swim. She ultimately turned her energies to ice hockey and was chosen as goalie for Team USA in the 2006 Winter Olympics. She made 50 saves in the Games as her team captured the bronze medal.

And did you know that the Supreme Court's current chief justice, John Roberts, has epilepsy?

That is quite a list! Clearly people with epilepsy come from all walks of life and have a variety of talents and skills. If epilepsy is a new diagnosis for you or a friend or family member, it is a lot to understand and consider. But you will be in the company of millions in the United States and millions more worldwide with the same condition.

Introduction to Seizures and Epilepsy

In the course of this book you will learn more in-depth information about seizures and epilepsy. Seizures can be quite varied in their appearance, from subtle symptoms known only to the person experiencing the seizure to very dramatic convulsions. In **Chapter 2** you will learn about each of the major seizure types and how they are divided into **focal** or **generalized seizures**, and acquire a common vocabulary to describe seizures that will be used throughout the rest of the book and to communicate with your medical team. A number of terms will be introduced that may be new to you, so I've included a Glossary at the end of the book. In case you don't remember what any of these words means, you can refer to the Glossary at any time.

Chapter 3 keeps a focus on the title of the book: how to navigate life with epilepsy. This section discusses a number of topics in which medical issues overlap with "real world" issues. Epilepsy can raise new concerns surrounding safety, including driving, so the chapter discusses ways to manage the balance of maintaining both independence and safety. Epilepsy's reach can extend into other aspects of life, including personal and work relationships; some common themes and ways of successfully navigating these areas are addressed.

As a brain disease, epilepsy commonly overlaps with other brain conditions. Many people have concerns about memory and thinking, mood, and anxiety. Special care is needed to manage these concerns in someone with epilepsy. Living well with epilepsy is a team approach, and the book includes suggestions for how family members and caregivers can most effectively participate to enhance the lives of people with epilepsy. **Chapter 3** closes with some practical tips for successful visits with your doctor in the clinic.

At the most fundamental level, epilepsy is a brain disorder, and it is helpful to know a little about the underlying brain science. The changes in the brain that lead to seizures can be very difficult even for scientists and epilepsy experts to fully understand. However, much has been learned in recent years about the scientific basis of epilepsy. The basic discussion in **Chapter 4** may make it easier to understand how seizures happen and how treatments to combat seizures are developed.

Chapter 5 addresses the causes and risks of developing epilepsy throughout the life span. While a disturbance in brain function is common to everyone with epilepsy, epilepsy has many different specific causes, making it different from some other conditions like Parkinson's disease, for example. Experts have argued that epilepsy is not really a single disease, but a collection of different disorders that have seizures as a common symptom. We will look at some of the most common causes and consider how each of these very different kinds of changes to the brain can cause seizures. Not all disturbances in brain function cause seizures. Among those that do, not all are equally likely to cause seizures. For example, some mild head injuries are not associated with an increased risk of seizures. Yet severe head injuries are very strongly connected to the later development of epilepsy. We will learn about risk factors for developing epilepsy, and which ones put someone at greatest risk. The causes of epilepsy are also very different for an infant, an adolescent, a middle-aged adult, and an elderly person.

With this information as background we will then turn to the central issues of diagnosis and treatment: what goes on when you go to the clinic and see your health care provider. Please note that for simplicity, I will more commonly use the term "doctor" instead of the more general but awkward term "health care provider." But it is important to point out that epilepsy is a complex disorder that often requires a team approach. While you will likely encounter a neurologist—a doctor specialized in the treatment of diseases of the brain, spinal cord, and nerves—there may often be other experts on the epilepsy team. Many epilepsy centers have nurses, nurse practitioners, or physician's assistants who provide care for people with epilepsy. In some cases, physicians in other, related fields may be involved in your care. These include **radiologists,** who interpret brain imaging tests. People with epilepsy may have concerns about memory and thinking, and some may see a **neuropsychologist**— a specialist in this area. It is not unusual for people with epilepsy also to have anxiety or depression, and a mental health professional (psychologist or psychiatrist) may also be part of the team. A few people for whom epilepsy surgery is the most effective treatment may see a neurosurgeon.

Chapter 6 looks at diagnosis. There is no simple blood test to determine whether someone has epilepsy. Instead, there is a process. If followed carefully, this process of carefully taking a medical history, performing a neurologic examination, and doing some limited supportive testing can reliably diagnose or exclude epilepsy in most people. In general, this process can take some time but does not involve painful or unusually uncomfortable procedures. For those in whom diagnosis is especially challenging, **Chapter 7** discusses specialized forms of diagnostic testing.

One of the biggest areas to cover is the treatment of epilepsy. Decision making about treatment is broken up into stages, and **Chapter 8** starts with the basics. Many people who have had a single seizure do not require treatment. Most people with epilepsy (recurrent, unprovoked seizures) *do* need some form of treatment. Before jumping into a discussion of medications, nonmedication approaches to reducing seizure risk will be considered—some lifestyle do's and don'ts that may help reduce the risk of seizures in everyone. Deciding if and when to start medication for seizures is addressed, as well as the other side of the coin—when and if it is safe to stop medications.

For nearly everyone with epilepsy, the first line of approach is medical therapy. Choice of an **antiepileptic drug**, or **AED** as they will be frequently called throughout this book, is critically important. More than 20 AEDs have been approved for use by the US Food and Drug Administration (FDA; see **Appendix 2** at the end of the book). This is good, because it means there are many options. Treatment can be individualized. If the first medication does not work or causes unacceptable side effects, there are many other choices. However, many choices can sometimes also lead to confusion. Where should you start? Your doctor will be the main person guiding you through the various medication options. But this process works best as a partnership between the person with epilepsy and the doctor.

To be an active partner, it is helpful to have reliable information about the various AED choices. Basic principles of AED selection will be covered in **Chapter 9**. Common side effects, drug interactions, and principles of lab monitoring are addressed in **Chapter 10**. **Appendix 2** at the end of the book will serve as a reference for some of the details about each AED.

For many people, initial AED trials are successful in stopping all seizures. With time, these individuals may resume most of their usual activities, including driving, and may only need to see their doctor infrequently. Unfortunately, for many others, things are more challenging. As many as one-third of people with epilepsy fail to achieve good seizure control with AED therapy. "Good" seizure control means complete control of seizures. It is clear from many studies that complete control of seizures is very different from having "only" one or two seizures per year. Those who are seizure free enjoy much better quality of life and sense of well-being. The goal is "seizure free, without side effects." But what if AED therapy doesn't achieve this objective?

Chapter 11 discusses surgical treatment of epilepsy. In general, surgical treatment of epilepsy is reserved for people whose seizures don't respond to reasonable AED trials. This does *not* mean that every medication in every combination must be tried before considering alternatives. That would take several lifetimes! In fact, we will see **medication-resistant epilepsy** can often be identified early. It is very important *not* to simply keep trying one medication after the other without success or to stay on the same AED and just accept having poor seizure control. One main message from **Chapter 11** is that treatments such as epilepsy surgery are not "last ditch" or "desperation" measures. Instead, epilepsy surgery should be thought of as simply a different approach that may be extremely effective even when AED therapy has failed.

Not everyone with medication-resistant epilepsy is a candidate for epilepsy surgery. **Chapter 12** explores the use of medical devices to treat seizures, diet therapy, and alternative therapies. Using medical devices to deliver neurostimulation—electrical therapy to the brain or connected nerves—offers a different option for people whose seizures are not controlled with AEDs, or in situations where side effects limit their dosing. Many people wish to try other treatment approaches that may be somewhat outside of the mainstream of Western medicine. These are often grouped together as **complementary and alternative medicine**, or **CAM**. Complementary therapies are those that might be used alongside conventional treatments, while alternative approaches might be used by some in place of conventional medicine. These therapies are widely used, and it is helpful to be aware of what is known and what is still not known about various CAM approaches. Some emerging areas of therapy are still being debated, and we will try to make some sense of any uncertainties.

Over the course of this book it will become clear that there is no "one size fits all" approach to epilepsy therapy. Certain groups of people with epilepsy, including women and older people, have unique issues and concerns, and treatment of some special populations is covered in **Chapter 13**.

Despite all of the work on the causes and treatments of epilepsy, not all aspects are fully understood and not everything can be presented as settled fact. In some areas, it would be easy to stir up a lively argument in a roomful of epilepsy experts! Recognizing this uncertainty, a few "debates in epilepsy" sections will appear throughout the book to give voice to these areas of ongoing debate.

It is a lot to cover, but if you take it a step at a time, it should be very manageable. As the Chinese proverb goes, "a journey of a thousand miles begins with a single step." Our first step will be to understand the terms "seizure" and "epilepsy."

Chapter 2

What Are Seizures and What Is Epilepsy?

In this chapter, we will first define seizures and epilepsy, and then go on to learn about the different types of seizures and how information about seizure types can be combined with other information to determine epilepsy syndromes. As we learned in Chapter 1, epilepsy diagnosis is about connecting the dots, and there is no single test that establishes the diagnosis.

General Introduction and Definitions

Before we get too far along, it is useful to review some basic definitions. A good starting point is to define the words **seizure** and **epilepsy**.

The International League Against Epilepsy (ILAE), the international group that supports the advancement of epilepsy education and patient care, defines a seizure as "manifestation(s) of epileptic (excessive and/or hypersynchronous), usually self-limited activity of neurons in the brain." That's a bit hard to interpret! Let's break this down, starting at the end of the definition.

A seizure is an event that begins in the brain. The brain cells, or **neurons**, normally communicate with each other in a very controlled way using small chemical and electrical signals. For example, your hands are getting a message from the motor areas of your brain that allow you to hold this book or e-reader.

The brain is organized so that most of the neurons live on the wrinkled surface of the brain: the **cortex** (see Figure 2–1).

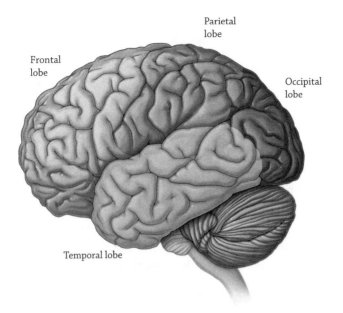

FIGURE 2-1 External surface of brain: cortex. Reproduced with permission from Caplan, L. *Navigating the Complexities of Stroke.* © American Academy of Neurology 2013.

When the cortex forms during early brain development, the neurons line up and connect in six layers. Underlying the cortex, or **gray matter**, is the **white matter**. The white matter is the wiring of the brain—the cables that connect the neurons to each other across different brain regions. These wires or cables also connect the neurons of the brain to the lower part of the brain—the brainstem—and also to the **spinal cord**. The brain is highly organized and specialized, with different areas controlling different functions and behaviors. Some areas in the occipital lobe are specialized for vision. Others in the frontal lobe are critical for motor (movement) function. Still others in the temporal lobe support short-term memory.

Under normal conditions, the activity of these neurons is precise and controlled, allowing each area to carry out its specific function efficiently. During a seizure this tightly controlled process is disrupted. Some think of a seizure as an electrical "storm" in the brain. The neurons involved in a seizure fire rapidly and may recruit their neighbors to do the same—so the activity is *excessive* and **hypersynchronous** (cells that don't normally fire together are all firing at the same time). The observable seizure is the *manifestation* of this abnormal brain activity—it is what results from the abnormal firing of neurons.

The manifestations of a seizure, including the symptoms (what the person with epilepsy experiences) and the signs (what observers see) can be very different depending on what group of neurons is involved with the seizure. More on this soon when we talk about seizure types.

Now that we have a basic definition of a seizure, what is epilepsy? The ILAE glossary definition of epilepsy is brief: "A chronic neurological condition characterized by recurrent epileptic seizures." This definition includes two key points:

- It is a chronic, or relatively long-lasting, condition
- It involves recurrent seizures

More detailed definitions also include the important idea that the recurrent seizures are "unprovoked." A **provoked seizure** results from a strong external provoking factor that can produce a seizure in someone who is not otherwise prone to having seizures. For example, if someone with diabetes takes too much insulin, their blood sugar could go very low, and this could trigger a seizure in someone with otherwise normal brain function. This distinction is important, because many people may have seizures in extreme circumstances, but that does not mean they have epilepsy. Thus anyone who has experienced two or more seizures that were *not* the direct result of a strong provoking factor (like too much insulin) has epilepsy.

In recent years, the definition has been modified to include two important ideas:

- Epilepsy implies a long-lasting risk for seizures
- Epilepsy carries consequences beyond the immediate effects of a seizure

Epilepsy is characterized by an *enduring predisposition* to generate seizures. Anyone can have a seizure in extreme circumstances, but someone with epilepsy has an ongoing tendency to have seizures *without* a strong provoking factor. Many experts believed that if this "enduring predisposition to generate seizures" could be established, epilepsy could be diagnosed following only a single seizure. As of 2014, this concept has been accepted as part of the definition of epilepsy. Most people will still be diagnosed with epilepsy after having more than one unprovoked seizure. But it is now possible to make the diagnosis earlier—after a single seizure—if there is a high risk of recurrence.

The second change recognizes that the effects of epilepsy extend beyond the seizures themselves. The proposed change states that epilepsy has "neurobiologic, cognitive, psychological, and social consequences." This recognizes what most people with epilepsy already know: Epilepsy is more than seizures. It may affect memory function and mood, and it may change how that person functions in society.

Ralph is 54 years old and has had diabetes since age 6, requiring daily insulin injections. Three years ago his dose of insulin was adjusted. His blood sugar dropped dangerously low, and he became confused and had a witnessed seizure. His insulin dose was adjusted further, but two weeks later he had food poisoning with nausea and vomiting for 48 hours. His blood sugar again dropped very low, and he had his second observed seizure.

His family might wonder: Does Ralph have epilepsy? He has clearly had two seizures, but these were both provoked by his very low blood sugar. Anyone with extremely low blood sugar can have a seizure. And since he does not have an "enduring predisposition to generate seizures" under normal circumstances, he does not have epilepsy.

> Jennifer is 40 years old and had been healthy until she had an observed seizure in the grocery store, without any apparent trigger. While going through the checkout, she stopped responding to the clerk, stared off into the distance, and made repetitive lip-smacking movements. When this ended she was very confused and did not know where she was or that the person standing next to her was her husband. Her husband recalled hearing her make the same lip-smacking sounds at night but thought it was just a "sleep thing" and didn't think to seek medical care.

Does Jennifer have epilepsy? She had an unprovoked seizure in the grocery store, and in retrospect, this was not her first seizure. She has had recurrent, unprovoked seizures and thus has epilepsy.

> Max is a successful 60-year-old businessman. He has inappropriately been using alcohol to manage stress, and after work most days he has six to eight alcoholic drinks, and sometimes more on the weekends. On two occasions when he decided to quit alcohol abruptly, he became shaky and confused and on both occasions had a single brief seizure.

Does Max have epilepsy? He has a problem with substance abuse (alcohol), and has had two seizures provoked by alcohol withdrawal.

If his substance abuse can be successfully treated, he should not have an "enduring predisposition to generate seizures." He had provoked seizures, but does not have epilepsy.

> Martha is 78 years old and has several health problems, including a history of heart attacks, irregular heart rhythm, and a history of a small stroke (blockage of blood flow to a small part of the brain causing minor but permanent injury). Her friends in her church group and her daughter have both seen her experience brief seizures without any apparent trigger.

Does Martha have epilepsy? Yes; Martha has had two unprovoked seizures and by definition has epilepsy. We'll learn more in later chapters about the causes of epilepsy, but in her age group, the history of stroke was probably the reason she developed epilepsy. In my experience, people in Martha's age group are often surprised to hear that they have epilepsy. For some people, the term "epilepsy" conjures up a specific image—for example, of a child with developmental disabilities and seizures. However, as we will see, adults over age 65 are the largest group with new-onset epilepsy.

Seizure Types

Entire books could be and have been written about seizure types. The goal for this book is to give you a basic understanding of the main ways that seizures are classified. This will provide a common language to describe seizures throughout the rest of the book and can help facilitate discussions with your doctor. Seizures are described by the behavior that happens during the seizure itself, called the **ictal** period, as well as by the immediate aftereffects of the seizure, known as the **postictal** period. "Ictal" is another word for seizure.

Experts have argued for years about the best way to classify seizure types. Some experts are "lumpers" who try to group common seizure types together and who focus on shared features; others are "splitters" who focus more on the differences between different seizure types. I have tried to steer a middle course between these two extremes. I will strive to explain clearly the major seizure types while avoiding getting bogged down in excessive detail. I hope that by the end of this section, you will be familiar with the terms for common seizure types and how they relate to each other.

Seizure Types: Focal and Generalized

Seizure types can be divided into two major groups. First, there are seizures that begin in a particular part of the brain: **focal** or **partial** seizures. Second, there are other seizure types that essentially start in the whole brain (or at least both halves of the brain) at once: **generalized seizures**. As we will see, this division is not perfect. Some seizures may not clearly fit one or the other pattern. A focal seizure can spread to later involve the whole brain. "Generalized" seizures, if studied carefully, probably don't really start in the whole brain at the same time. Still, this broad division into focal and generalized seizures is a useful way to organize seizure types. This distinction between focal and generalized seizure types will also be important to keep in mind when we discuss treatment.

Focal (or Partial) Seizures

As just mentioned, focal or partial seizures begin in a particular area of the brain. You will likely hear the terms "focal" and "partial" used interchangeably; however, most experts prefer the term "focal" because there is really no such thing as a partial seizure—either you have a seizure or you don't; there is nothing "partial" about it. Sometimes the focus may truly be a single spot in the brain—a very well-defined focus. At other times the focus may be a slightly larger region of the brain, what scientists call a "network" of connected brain cells.

There are three basic types of focal seizures:

- Simple partial seizures
- Complex partial seizures
- Secondarily generalized tonic-clonic seizures

Although we divide focal seizures into these three groups, they are closely related to one another. The division into the three types is based on how much the seizure spreads from the original focus (see Figure 2–2). A seizure may begin as a simple partial seizure, then spread from the original focus to cause a complex partial seizure, and in some cases it may ultimately spread to the whole brain, causing a secondarily generalized tonic-clonic (also a called "convulsive" or "grand mal" seizure).

    a. A **simple partial seizure** remains relatively confined to the area where the seizure began. The term "simple" refers to the fact that consciousness is not affected. The person

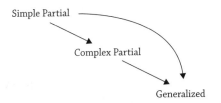

FIGURE 2-2 The spectrum of focal seizures.

experiencing the seizure is fully awake and aware of what is happening and can generally remember the whole event later. The actual symptoms and signs of the seizure can be very different depending on where in the brain the seizure originates (Box 2–1).

BOX 2-1 Common Types of Simple Partial Seizures

- Motor
  - Clonic (jerking or twitching of a body part)
  - Versive (head or eye turning to one side)
  - Dystonic (holding a body part in an odd, fixed posture)
- Sensory
  - Touch (tingling or "pins-and-needles" sensation that may spread)
  - Visual (colors, shapes, or formed images)
  - Auditory (buzzing, loud sound)
  - Smells ("olfactory hallucinations")
  - Taste (odd, often foul tastes)
- Autonomic
  - A rising feeling in the belly (feeling like moving in an elevator)
  - Flushing or sweating
  - "Goosebumps"
  - Eyes getting bigger (dilated pupils)
- Psychic
  - Fear sensation (can seem like a panic attack, but usually shorter)
  - Déjà vu (feeing like new things are very familiar or that you have been doing or did what you are doing before)
  - Jamais vu (feeling like everything in the environment is unfamiliar)

Sometimes the term "aura" is used to describe the beginning of a seizure, especially when the seizure begins with symptoms that are only internally experienced and not observable by others. The word "aura" comes from the Greek word meaning "breeze" and can be a subtle but recognizable feeling that passes over a person beginning to experience a seizure. In popular culture, the term "aura" has sometimes been used to describe a visual glow or outline around objects as seen by someone with psychic powers, but this is a very different use of the term and not a typical experience of people with epilepsy. The aura is not separate from the seizure but describes the beginning symptoms in someone who retains full awareness; it is really another term for a simple partial seizure. It represents the limited symptoms caused by a seizure confined to a focal part of the brain.

b. A **complex partial seizure** (see Figure 2–2) implies that there has been further spread of the seizure from the original focus, usually involving at least a limited part of both halves, or **hemispheres,** of the brain. The term "complex" refers to the fact that consciousness is impaired during the seizure. The person experiencing the seizure often appears conscious— he or she may not fall to the ground or have closed eyes as with a fainting spell—but is not able to respond normally to the environment and his or her memory will be impaired. A person having a complex partial seizure usually has his or her eyes open and may continue to stand or sit upright, but may stare or have a vacant or dull look in the eyes. The spouses or friends of several of my patients have described this as "lights on, but no one is home."

Complex partial seizures are often accompanied by **automatisms**. Automatisms are automatic behaviors that occur during complex partial seizures. Some of these may appear semipurposeful— arranging items on a table or manipulating a cellphone that was held in the hand at the start of the seizure—but on closer examination, the movements don't usually accomplish anything. The items are rearranged on the table randomly. The buttons of the cellphone are pressed, but in a random string of digits. An individual may have his or her own personal set of automatisms that friends or loved ones may recognize as distinctive. "Whenever I hear him repetitively tapping on something, I know a seizure is happening," says Lenore, the wife of one of my patients.

Box 2–2 lists some of the most common forms of automatisms.

Speech and language are often affected in a complex partial seizure. Language is a specialized function that is usually located in the left hemisphere of the brain, sometimes called the *dominant hemisphere*. In a few people—more commonly in left-handed people—language function may be located on the opposite side. For these individuals, the right hemisphere is their dominant hemisphere. Thus, if a seizure begins in the dominant hemisphere, speech is more prominently affected. If seizures start in the nondominant hemisphere, or away from language areas, speech may be preserved during complex partial seizures, although the content of the speech may not make sense, and the ability to understand and follow directions may be affected.

BOX 2-2 Common Automatisms

- Chewing
- Lip smacking
- Repetitive swallowing
- Fumbling with objects
- Picking at clothing
- Repeated vocalizations
- Complex movements such as clapping, pointing, waving arms, gesturing

Following a complex partial seizure, there is often a period of confusion. The period of time after a seizure when the person (and his or her brain) is recovering from a seizure is called the *postictal period*. Following a seizure the person is said to be in the **postictal state**. Sometimes people will say that someone is "postictal" for short. This period of confusion and disorientation often lasts for seconds to a few minutes. During this period of confusion, people may act in ways that are out of character for them. They may be more aggressive or combative, especially if someone tries to hold or restrain them. It can be very challenging for friends or family members to know what to do. They have to be concerned about safety, as someone could wander off and get into trouble in the postictal state. One of my patients wandered out into the snow barefoot and contracted mild frostbite. Another ended up in a neighbor's house in a very confused state. Maintaining safety in the postictal state is of paramount importance. At the same time, trying to restrain someone too aggressively can provoke a more physical response. It can be difficult to steer the middle course: to reassure, reorient, and guide the individual away from danger without being too physically confrontational.

Parts of the brain fire very rapidly during a seizure, and these areas may temporarily shut down or not function very well as the brain recovers, or resets itself, after the seizure. Brain areas nearest the seizure onset may be most exhausted and may take the longest to recover. Temporary symptoms may be related to the dysfunction of that brain area. The most common example is temporary weakness. This temporary weakness is sometimes called a **Todd's paralysis** (named for the nineteenth-century physician Robert Bentley Todd who described it), and results from seizures that involve parts of the brain that control muscle or motor function. Many people know that the left side of the body is mostly controlled by the right brain, and vice versa. Thus a seizure that begins in the motor areas of the left brain may result in temporary weakness of the right body after the seizure has ended: a Todd's paralysis. The weakness usually lasts for seconds to minutes and quickly returns to normal. It is very different from a stroke, which causes permanent brain injury, but can look similar for a few moments. Seizures beginning in nonmotor parts of the brain can cause different temporary problems as the brain recovers. For example, seizures that start in visual areas of the brain are less common but can result in temporary problems with vision following the seizure.

During complex partial seizures, other normal functions can be affected, including bladder control. For some people, this can be one of the most distressing symptoms of a seizure.

Finally, when recovery from the complex partial seizure is complete, people who have experienced a seizure may have no recall of the seizure at all. They have amnesia for that entire period or are said to be *amnestic* for everything that happened. This can be so profound that the individual may not believe that a seizure really happened. Understandably, more than once this has been the source of an argument between spouses.

c. A **secondarily generalized tonic-clonic (2°GTC)** seizure occurs when a focal seizure spreads fully to involve the whole brain. This seizure type may begin with a simple partial seizure (or aura) and progress to confusion (a complex partial seizure) before *secondarily* generalizing. Alternatively, the spread from the original seizure focus may be so rapid that the early symptoms go unnoticed.

The *tonic* and *clonic* phases define a secondarily generalized tonic-clonic seizure. In the tonic phase of this seizure type, the muscles contract or become rigid. Sometimes this can be seen first in the side of the body opposite the seizure focus in the brain. An arm or leg or both may stiffen, and the head may turn forcefully to one side, with the muscles of the face pulling in the same direction. Eventually both sides of the body stiffen, usually with the limbs extended in a straight, stiffened posture. The breathing muscles usually contract forcefully also, often forcing air out of the lungs causing a sound that is recognizable and that is sometimes called an "ictal cry."

During this tonic phase, which may often last for 10–30 seconds, the muscles remain stiff and no breathing can occur. This may cause the lips or fingers to temporarily appear blue or dark in color.

Next, there is a transition to the clonic phase. In the clonic phase of a seizure, periodic brief jerking or "clonic" movements occur. These movements are usually easiest to see in the limbs, but they may affect the whole body. Typically, the clonic movements are small and rapid at first but become larger and slower in frequency over time before finally stopping.

The postictal phase following a 2°GTC can be more profound than after a complex partial seizure. Initially the person who experienced the seizure may appear deeply asleep. There may be snoring-like breathing sounds. Often saliva production has increased during the seizure, and this period carries the greatest risk for breathing it into the lungs. This is called aspiration and can lead to lung infections (pneumonia). Positioning the patient on his or her side is the best protection from aspiration. Seizure first aid will be discussed in detail in Chapter 3. After this most intense postictal period, a further period of confusion, amnesia, and disorientation, as described earlier for complex partial seizures, often follows. Tongue biting is another common symptom of a 2°GTC, which is often discovered following the seizure.

By now we have seen that focal seizures can be simple partial, complex partial, or secondarily generalized, depending on the degree of spread from the original seizure focus (Table 2–1). In real life, seizures may not fall neatly into these categories. It may be hard to judge whether, or how much, consciousness is impaired. Some have focused on these uncertainties and have suggested that this system of classification be abandoned. However, it is still the system that is most commonly in use, and the one that you will probably use to communicate with your doctor.

TABLE 2-1 Focal Seizures

Seizure Type	Defining Feature	Signs and Symptoms
Simple partial	Preserved awareness	Depends on location of seizure focus in the brain
Complex partial	Confusion, altered awareness of environment	Confusion, limited ability to interact, often automatic behaviors or automatisms
Secondarily generalized tonic-clonic	Tonic (stiffening) and clonic (jerking) movements	Unconsciousness, tonic and clonic motor behavior

Generalized Seizure Types

Next, we will turn to a description of the other major group of seizure types: generalized-from-onset seizures. In contrast to focal-onset seizures, this group of seizures does not have a well-defined focus. Because they involve both sides of the brain from onset, most of them cause rapid loss of conscious awareness without any warning symptoms. The most common generalized seizure types include:

- Absence seizures
- Atypical absence seizures
- Generalized tonic-clonic seizures
- Myoclonic seizures
- Tonic seizures
- Atonic seizures

Absence Seizures

These are brief seizures that are most often seen in children. In some people, absence seizures can persist into adolescence or adulthood. They used to be called "petit mal" seizures. They consist of a sudden loss of awareness or disconnection from the environment. There is usually an abrupt behavioral arrest ("freezing," but no falls), followed by rapid return to normal after five to 10 seconds. Unlike a complex partial seizure (see previous section), there is no period of postictal confusion. Someone who has experienced an absence seizure can generally pick up right where he or she left off and is usually unaware that a seizure has occurred. Absence seizures often occur repeatedly, many times per day. Children with absence seizures may be labeled as "inattentive" in school because they are missing many small parts of the day. Occasionally, other features can be seen, such as subtle blinking or small hand or mouth movements. These are sometimes seen in absence seizures of longer duration.

Atypical Absence Seizures

"Atypical" absence seizures are different from the usual absence seizures in several ways. They often last longer than a typical absence seizure (20 to 30 seconds or more). There may be a gradual onset and offset, and a person experiencing an atypical absence seizure may seem partially responsive during the event. Often this seizure type is seen in people who have other seizure types and who have some degree of intellectual disability.

Generalized Tonic-clonic Seizures

This seizure type involves sudden loss of consciousness with the same tonic (muscle stiffening) and then clonic (muscle jerking) components described previously with a secondarily generalized tonic-clonic seizure. The difference lies in the seizure onset. Here the seizure begins abruptly and simultaneously in both halves of the brain, resulting in tonic and clonic phases of a seizure that affect both sides of the body more or less equally. This is different from the *secondarily generalized* tonic-clonic seizure, which begins focally and then spreads to the whole brain. However, if you walk into the room when someone is having a generalized tonic-clonic seizure, it may not be possible to tell if it was generalized from onset or whether the seizure was the result of secondary generalization from a focus. Other observations or tests may help make that distinction.

We will see that the distinction can be an important. It can determine choice of treatments and understanding what to expect in the future (prognosis).

Myoclonic Seizures

Myoclonic seizures are very brief sudden jerks of the muscles. Commonly, myoclonic seizures consist of twitches or jerks of the arms and upper body, but they may also affect the trunk, legs, or face. They may occur as a sudden isolated twitch that lasts for a fraction of a second, but they also often occur in clusters of repetitive brief twitches over a period of a few seconds. Usually the person experiencing a myoclonic seizure is fully awake and aware of what is happening. With a longer cluster there may be a brief loss of awareness. Strong myoclonic seizures that affect the trunk or legs could lead to a fall and injury, but most of the time this does not happen.

Often people don't think of these brief jerking movements as seizures.

Rosa had her first generalized tonic-clonic seizure at age 16. When her neurologist specifically asked about symptoms of myoclonic seizures, he discovered that she had actually been having myoclonic seizures since age 14. She had just thought of herself as "clumsy" when her myoclonic jerks would cause her to drop something. She did not connect her myoclonus seizures with her epilepsy until her neurologist specifically asked her about brief jerking movements.

It is also important to know that not all myoclonus is epileptic myoclonus. In other words, the same movement of myoclonus may not be related to epilepsy in many people. Myoclonus may also be produced by metabolic disturbances, certain medications, other brain diseases, and certain genetic conditions, just to name a few.

The movements can look the same as myoclonic seizures, but the cause is different.

Some myoclonus can even be normal. Many of us have had the experience of having a sudden jerking movement when falling asleep, especially if we are very tired. That is myoclonus! It is a specific type sometimes called sleep myoclonus or "hypnic jerks." It is normal. Another form of myoclonus we are all probably familiar with is hiccups. Hiccups represent a myoclonic jerk of the diaphragm, one of the muscles above the belly that aids breathing.

Drop Seizures (Tonic Seizures and Atonic Seizures)

Tonic and atonic seizures are sometimes grouped together and called **drop seizures** because they can both cause sudden falls. They both disrupt the brain systems that keep us standing. With a tonic seizure, there is a sudden stiffening of muscles throughout the body. In contrast, an atonic seizure produces a sudden loss of muscle tone. Both types of drop seizures usually begin in childhood and are often seen in people who have additional other seizure types and intellectual disability.

Both types of seizures can lead to sudden falls. The sudden muscle stiffening with a tonic seizure can cause a sudden fall if the person is standing. People witnessing a tonic seizure often say the person seemed to "topple like a tree." In an atonic seizure, there is often a sudden collapse to the ground without any protective reflexes. The appearance of an atonic seizure can be very subtle—a quick head drop when seated—but if standing, sudden falls can result in severe injury. Both tonic and atonic seizures can be frequent and difficult to control with medications.

Falls from drop seizures can result in severe injuries such as bone fractures, including fractures of the skull and facial bones. The usual reflexes that help us land more safely when we fall are absent. Since the onset of drop seizures is very abrupt, it is hard to anticipate them or always be prepared to catch someone when the seizure starts. It is common for people with this seizure type to wear protective gear such as a hockey helmet. Some people become mostly confined to a wheelchair because of the very high risk of injury.

You now have an understanding of the main seizure types that can occur. Understanding seizure types is important to the diagnosis and understanding of epilepsy. But the process doesn't stop there. When knowledge of the seizure type is combined with other information, more powerful information emerges. This leads us to the concept of **epilepsy syndromes**.

Epilepsy Syndromes

Now that we have a basic understanding of seizure types, we can turn to a discussion of epilepsy syndromes. Some of the details may be more important to your doctor than to you. But the concept of a syndrome, and a story to illustrate why it is important, are worth spending a little time on.

A syndrome is a group of features that usually occur together and characterize a particular condition. Seizure types are important in defining an epilepsy syndrome, but the syndrome also integrates other information. This includes the medical and epilepsy history, such as the age that seizures began, the time of day that seizures occur, and their frequency and severity. If other family members are known to have epilepsy, this information is included, because some epilepsy syndromes are caused by changes in genes. Also considered is assessment of the cause of the epilepsy (if known), risk factors for epilepsy (see Chapter 5), and findings on testing such as **electroencephalogram (EEG)** and **magnetic resonance imaging (MRI)** scan results (see Chapter 7).

The power of going beyond seizure types to understanding the epilepsy syndrome is twofold. First, specific epilepsy syndromes may have an expected prognosis or "natural course." Understanding the syndrome can help everyone know what to expect in the future and help answer a lot of common questions: Can this epilepsy be outgrown? Will lifelong treatment for seizures be needed, or is it likely that antiepileptic medications could be safely discontinued in the future? Second, knowledge of the epilepsy syndrome can help predict responsiveness to specific treatments or antiepileptic drugs, and can be used to guide therapy.

We opened the book with the story of Sebastian, who was diagnosed with epilepsy at age 17 when he had his first generalized tonic-clonic seizure. With more questioning, his doctor learned that he also had been experiencing myoclonic seizures for at least 2 years, but these were subtle and were not thought of as seizures at the time. Although it was helpful for Sebastian's doctor to understand the seizure types, that information alone didn't help answer many of Sebastian's questions. Would he develop very severe epilepsy that would substantially change the course of his life? Would he quickly gain control of the seizures and return to his usual activities? As we will see in the next several chapters, getting more information to define Sebastian's epilepsy syndrome can make a big difference.

His neurologist asked more questions about his family and personal medical history. She did more testing, including an EEG and MRI of the brain. When all of this information was put together, she could give Sebastian a specific epilepsy syndrome diagnosis. Sebastian has an epilepsy syndrome called **juvenile myoclonic epilepsy**, or **JME**. This epilepsy syndrome diagnosis is much more powerful than a simple description of the seizure types. It tells us that the odds are good that Sebastian's seizures will be controlled with medication. It also predicts that he will likely need to be on lifelong therapy to prevent seizures. Neither of these could have been predicted from the seizure type alone.

Knowledge of the epilepsy syndrome may also help guide therapy. It may suggest a medication, or a group of medications, that might work best to treat the epilepsy. It may predict when medications are unlikely to work, and when we should consider other methods of treating epilepsy, such as epilepsy surgery or use of medical devices.

Charlotte had experienced seizures as a child that came under good control with medications. She was able to come off of medications for several years, but then her seizures came back at age 12 and proved to be difficult to control. Her seizure types included simple partial, complex partial, and rare secondarily generalized tonic-clonic seizures. With additional questioning and testing she was found to have a specific syndrome called **mesial temporal sclerosis (MTS)**.

Much is known about the syndrome of mesial temporal sclerosis. A known group of medications is available to treat people who have MTS. However, we also know that this syndrome is often resistant to treatment with medication, and seizures may persist despite therapy. Fortunately, we also know that this syndrome responds very well to epilepsy surgery. Identification and surgical removal of the seizure focus can lead to seizure freedom even when medications have had little benefit.

Many epilepsy syndromes are specific to young children and are not a focus of this book. One common childhood syndrome that can persist into adolescence and adulthood is **Lennox-Gastaut syndrome (LGS)**.

Nate was diagnosed with Lennox-Gastaut syndrome in early childhood. He had a cluster of different seizure types, including drop seizures, which are typical for this syndrome, as well as generalized tonic-clonic seizures and atypical absences. His intellectual development was impaired, and his EEG (brain wave) test showed a typical pattern for LGS.

Lennox-Gastaut syndrome is often associated with severe and difficult-to-control seizures. The *syndrome diagnosis* of LGS is not the same as the *cause* of Nate's epilepsy. A number of different underlying brain conditions can produce the pattern of features seen in LGS. In up to a quarter of cases, no definite underlying cause can be identified. However, it is the *syndrome* pattern that guides decision making for therapy and expectations for prognosis.

Other childhood syndromes such as childhood absence epilepsy and benign epilepsy with centrotemporal spikes (BECTS) are milder, and we can tell these children and parents that they are likely to "outgrow" their epilepsy as they mature into adolescence and early adulthood.

There are too many specific epilepsy syndromes to list them all here. To add to the complexity, epilepsy experts are continually rethinking and reorganizing the syndromes based on new information that comes to light, and diving into all of the details and rules for how different syndromes are determined is not likely to be helpful for our purposes. For reference, Box 2–3 shows a list of some of the named epilepsy syndromes that appear at different ages, as modified from the organization that has taken the lead on defining these syndromes, the International League Against Epilepsy (ILAE).

Even this partial list can get quickly overwhelming! The details are less important for our purposes. Many times it can be hard to know the exact epilepsy syndrome for an individual. Sometimes we can identify a general syndrome category, and other times we can identify a specific named epilepsy syndrome.

For now, let's try to just keep in mind the *concept* of an epilepsy syndrome. An epilepsy syndrome goes beyond a simple description of the seizure type(s) and brings in other information that can be a powerful guide to choosing treatment and understanding prognosis.

BOX 2-3 Epilepsy Syndromes

Epilepsy Syndromes Usually Beginning in Newborns

Benign familial neonatal epilepsy (BFNE)
Early myoclonic encephalopathy (EME)
Ohtahara syndrome

Epilepsy Syndromes Usually Beginning in Infants

West syndrome
Myoclonic epilepsy in infancy (MEI)
Benign infantile epilepsy
Benign familial infantile epilepsy
Dravet syndrome

Epilepsy Syndromes Usually Beginning in Childhood

Panayiotopoulos syndrome
Epilepsy with myoclonic atonic (previously called astatic) seizures
Benign epilepsy with centrotemporal spikes (BECTS)
Autosomal-dominant nocturnal frontal lobe epilepsy (ADNFLE)
Late-onset childhood occipital epilepsy (Gastaut type)
Epilepsy with myoclonic absences
Lennox-Gastaut syndrome
Epileptic encephalopathy with continuous spike-and-wave during sleep (CSWS)
Landau-Kleffner syndrome (LKS)
Childhood absence epilepsy (CAE)

(Continued)

BOX 2-3 (Continued)

*Epilepsy Syndromes Usually Beginning
in Adolescence or Adulthood*

Juvenile absence epilepsy (JAE)
Juvenile myoclonic epilepsy (JME)
Epilepsy with generalized tonic-clonic seizures alone
Progressive myoclonus epilepsies (PME)

*Epilepsy Syndromes Seen in Adults That May
Also Start Earlier in Life*

Reflex epilepsies
Mesial temporal lobe epilepsy with hippocampal sclerosis
(MTLE with HS)
Focal epilepsy related to a specific cause
Malformations of cortical development
Tumor
Infection
Trauma
Blood vessel malformations
Stroke
Many others

Status Epilepticus

Before we leave seizure types and syndromes, it is useful to touch on one additional area: **status epilepticus**. This is not a distinct seizure type, but instead refers to seizures of any type that are especially prolonged. As we have seen, virtually all seizures stop by themselves. Some seizures end within seconds, and almost all within a minute or two. Rarely, the normal "stop signs" for seizures fail, and seizures can be uncontrolled and prolonged. Status epilepticus describes a situation in which a seizure lasts 30 minutes or longer. It can also refer to a series of seizures over a period of 30 minutes or more in which there is no recovery between seizures.

The 30-minute mark is mostly for the purpose of defining status epilepticus. Seizures that are likely to become status epilepticus can often be identified much earlier, allowing doctors to start treating people sooner. In Chapter 3, in the section "Safety and Seizure First Aid," we discuss a 5-minute rule. Any seizure that has continued for 5 minutes may likely be destined to progress to status epilepticus, and emergency treatment should be started.

If you or your loved one has epilepsy, this is the most important point in this section: Status epilepticus is a medical emergency that is potentially life threatening. People with status epilepticus have the best outcomes when it is treated early, so it is critically important to be ready with a response—usually calling 911, but sometimes having at-home acute seizure therapies (Chapter 13) that might help avoid a trip to the hospital and status epilepticus.

Although rare, any seizure type can be prolonged and lead to status epilepticus. The most concerning type is convulsive status epilepticus: prolonged generalized tonic-clonic activity. Prolonged convulsive seizures can put numerous body systems at risk. These include muscle breakdown that can injure the kidneys, elevated body temperature, heart rhythm disturbances, decreases in blood pressure, and disruption of metabolism. In addition, prolonged seizures can injure the brain. With typical brief seizures, the brain essentially "resets" itself following a seizure, after a period of recovery. With extended seizures in status epilepticus, there is greater concern that the prolonged seizures could lead to brain injury that is irreversible.

Estimates are that 60,000 to 150,000 episodes of status epilepticus occur every year in the United States. The causes of status epilepticus may fall into one of two groups: those with reversible causes and those related to acute brain injury.

Many people with reversible causes of status epilepticus have a previously known history of epilepsy. Often some event (for example, stopping their antiepileptic drugs or illness with fever) triggers an unusually prolonged seizure. Status epilepticus can also be triggered by drug and alcohol use or withdrawal or sudden changes in blood chemistry caused by other illness. If the status epilepticus can be treated early, the outlook is generally favorable since the cause is often reversible.

The second group includes those in whom the status epilepticus is caused by an acute brain injury. Many of these people do not have a previous history of epilepsy. Examples include stroke, traumatic brain injury, and brain infections (for example, meningitis or encephalitis). In these situations the status epilepticus is sometimes harder to control and the brain condition that is the cause of the status may be dangerous and not fully reversible. Here the outlook is more guarded.

Taking care to follow instructions on AED dosing can help reduce the risk of status epilepticus. Missing AED doses or stopping medication abruptly is one of the risk factors for status. If you are at high risk for status epilepticus, there are some medications that can be used at home in the event of repetitive or prolonged seizures. These medications are discussed in Chapter 13.

Chapter 3

Living with and Managing Epilepsy

This may be the most practical of all of the chapters in this book. In this chapter, we will look at best practices for seizure first aid. We'll then go on to talk about some of the common issues where epilepsy can affect day-to-day life, including driving, the workplace, and relationships. Because epilepsy is a brain condition, it may affect thinking and memory abilities, mood, and psychological health. Sometimes these areas can affect quality of life as much as or more than seizures, so it is a very important area to be knowledgeable about. The chapter closes with some practical tips on how to make interactions with your neurologist as productive as possible.

Safety and Seizure First Aid

Everyone who knows someone with epilepsy should learn the basics of seizure first aid. In this section we will focus on first aid for a generalized tonic-clonic seizure, although some of the principles can also apply to other seizure types.

There is nothing complicated about seizure first aid. With knowledge of a few basic principles, you will be prepared. However, if you have ever tried to help someone having a seizure, you likely found it stressful. Which brings us to the first principle: Take a deep breath, and stay calm! Many people find it helpful to watch someone deliver seizure first aid before they are called on to do so. There is an excellent video at http://www.epilepsy.com/firstaid that walks you through the process.

Preventing injury is a guiding principle, and some steps are common sense:

- Try to prevent a fall.
- On the ground, try to cushion the head with a jacket or other soft object if possible.
- If you can, check the time so you have an idea of how long the seizure lasts.

Positioning is the next step:

- If possible, the ideal position for a person having a seizure is on his or her side. Excessive saliva can be produced during a seizure, and this position will ensure that it does not enter the airway. Try to turn the person to his or her side, but do not force this—sometimes the arms are very stiff during a seizure and it is possible to cause an injury (such as a dislocated shoulder) by using too much force.

There are a few important "don'ts" also:

- Don't try to hold the person down or keep him or her from shaking.
- Do not attempt to put anything in the mouth of a person having a seizure. This can be quite dangerous and instead of helping, may end up injuring teeth or lead to the person biting the object and swallowing or choking on it.

If the seizure is brief (less than a minute or two), stay with the person during the recovery period. Be prepared that people are often quite confused after a seizure. A calm, reassuring voice is your best tool. Don't try to restrain someone following a seizure. That is likely to provoke a combative response, even in a normally calm individual. The exception might be if the confused person is headed for potential injury (for example, trying to wander out into traffic). Calm, clear instructions and a firm but not forcible guiding hand is the best strategy.

When is it important to call 911 and get emergency responders on the scene? There are several situations where this is best:

- A first seizure or a seizure in a person not known to you
- A seizure accompanied by injury or vomiting
- A seizure that lasts more than 5 minutes, or one in which the person is not beginning to wake up within 5 minutes
- Repeated seizures
- Seizures in someone who you have determined (for example, from a medical alert bracelet, or from observation) has another serious medical condition such as diabetes or pregnancy
- When in doubt, dial 911!

I want to assure you that it is really not too complicated if you have thought through things in advance. If you live with someone who has epilepsy, and especially if he or she has frequent tonic-clonic seizures, you might consider doing CPR training, for the rare instances when more resuscitation could be needed. Rescue breathing and CPR should not be done routinely in someone with a seizure—only in the rare instance where a seizure has stopped and the person does not resume breathing.

Navigating the Day-to-Day with Epilepsy

Driving

Driving is consistently identified as a leading concern for people with epilepsy. This is not surprising. In our society, driving is closely connected with a sense of independence. In many areas where public transportation is limited, it may be the only means of transportation for work and social activities.

There is general agreement that the privilege of driving must be balanced in some way with concerns about public safety. If a person has frequent seizures with loss of consciousness, he or she should not drive. If seizures are well controlled, either on or off antiepileptic drug (AED) therapy, driving should be permitted.

However, there is a substantial gray area where the determination of when it is safe to drive is more difficult. Driving laws add another layer of complexity to the medical decision about safe driving, and these laws vary substantially from state to state in the United States and among different countries. In the United States, a standard of being free of seizures with altered consciousness for 3 to 6 months is the most common. A useful resource is the Epilepsy Foundation's website, www.epilepsy.com, which has a state driving laws database at www.epilepsy.com/driving-laws.

Debates in Epilepsy: Driving and Seizure Reporting

In most states, people with epilepsy are asked to self-report seizures to the Department of Motor Vehicles (DMV). However, a few states still have provider-mandated reporting. This means doctors and other health care providers are legally required to report their patients' seizures to the state DMV.

Seizure reporting for the purposes of regulating licensure is controversial. There is fairly broad agreement that people having frequent seizures with impairment of consciousness should not drive. But either system of reporting (patient self-reporting or provider-mandated reporting) is potentially problematic. With patient self-reporting, people may be reluctant to report seizures because the consequence could be restriction or loss of driving privileges. Studies have in fact confirmed a substantial rate of underreporting among people with seizures.

(Continued)

(Continued)

However, health care provider reporting of seizures is not the simple solution it might seem. Professionals who care for people with epilepsy have expressed great concern about provider-mandated reporting. The concern is that the doctor will be put in a "policing" role. This role may discourage people from reporting seizure events to their doctors, leading to misguided epilepsy treatment. All systems of seizure reporting are imperfect. But because of the conflict created by provider-mandated reporting, most of the major medical and neurology societies oppose this system of reporting.

Many studies have examined the actual risk of driving in people with epilepsy. How great is the risk of accidents from seizures? Good quality data are hard to come by. It appears that the risk of accidents is somewhat higher in people with epilepsy—but perhaps not dramatically so. Epilepsy is a highly visible condition, and when a seizure occurs while driving, the results can be dramatic. This draws attention to the problem and might lead some to propose very strict rules. However, compared with other medical conditions in which driving is less routinely restricted, such as diabetes, heart disease, and alcoholism, the risk for driving accidents in epilepsy is equivalent or often lower. Most studies suggest that accident rates in healthy teenagers is much higher than for people with epilepsy.

In addition, not all seizures are the same. Some provisions may be made for people with certain seizure types. Those with a reliable, longstanding pattern of seizures *only* arising from sleep may be permitted to drive, even if their sleep-onset seizures are not completely controlled. Occasionally, people with a reliable and prolonged aura may be permitted to drive, even when seizures are incompletely controlled. There may be circumstances when a breakthrough seizure does not need to trigger a prolonged driving restriction. One example could be a seizure in association with an illness with severe nausea and vomiting that limits the ability to take AED therapy for a short period of time. If the seizures were previously well controlled on AED therapy, there would be every expectation that seizure control would resume when AED dosing resumes, and an extended period of observation to confirm seizure freedom may not be needed.

Because of its importance and controversial aspects, driving and epilepsy can be a highly emotional topic. Guidelines and laws should not selectively restrict driving in people with epilepsy relative to drivers with other at-risk medical conditions. The best decisions can be made on a foundation of solid information. Further data on the specific risks of different seizure types are needed. Good-quality studies can guide the optimal balance between protecting public safety and individual freedom.

Work

Many people with epilepsy are able to find and maintain fulfilling work. For many people, work provides structure, a sense of purpose, and of course, financial rewards.

If your seizure control is incomplete, it is worthwhile to think carefully about what kind of job would be most successful for you. Vocational counseling to match your skills and needs to a well-suited job can be very helpful. Avoiding jobs in which driving plays a central role may be an important consideration. Jobs with more flexible hours, such as being a consultant or a website designer, are sometimes desirable. Certain jobs, especially those that connect to public safety, have specific rules governing hiring of people with epilepsy. Examples include truck driver, airplane pilot, and air traffic controller, among others.

People with epilepsy are potentially subject to discrimination when seeking jobs. The issue of employment is closely tied to legal issues. The guiding legal regulations were written into the Americans with Disabilities Act (ADA), passed in 1990. Briefly, the

ADA sets out rules for public and many private employers that prohibit discrimination against qualified job applicants or employees on the basis of disability. This law is similar to those that protect the rights of women and minorities.

To accomplish the goal of protecting qualified people with disabilities, the ADA contains a number of specific rules to guide the interactions between employers and employees. What can an employer ask about disability? What must an employee disclose? What reasonable accommodations must an employer make for a qualified employee with a disability?

These topics are covered extremely well and in detail by the Epilepsy Foundation. See Appendix 1 for additional information and the URL.

The Equal Employment Opportunity Commission (EEOC) is the government body charged with enforcing the provisions of the ADA. The Epilepsy Foundation website just referenced has links to guide those in need of EEOC support, and helpful information for locating an attorney who might be able to provide advice or representation on employment issues if needed.

Relationships

People with epilepsy face many of the same relationship challenges as people who do not have seizures. Life events occur that may stress and challenge relationships, and, in response, relationships may strengthen, change, or end. But people with epilepsy must navigate a number of unique issues that can affect relationships.

Some of these issues are connected to problems that are more common in people with epilepsy, and several of these are addressed in other sections of this book. Depression, anxiety, and other psychological challenges are common in epilepsy and can have a tremendous impact on relationships. The diagnosis and management of psychological issues in people with epilepsy is the subject of the next section of this chapter. Epilepsy and seizures can affect coworker relationships, as just discussed in the Work section. Sexual dysfunction, often directly related to epilepsy and its treatment, can also affect intimate relationships. Because of the connection to AED therapy, this issue is addressed with medication side effects in Chapter 10.

In addition, a number of epilepsy-specific influences can complicate (or enrich) relationships. Especially when it begins at a young age, epilepsy may potentially limit social opportunities and lead to greater than average social isolation. This isolation can have several potential sources. There may be a tendency to avoid social situations out of fear that a seizure might occur in public. Well-meaning parents may be overprotective of a child or teen with epilepsy. And unfortunately, the stigma still attached to epilepsy may lead some who are unfamiliar with or frightened by seizures to limit social and relationship contacts with people with epilepsy.

In the early periods of romantic relationships, or even friendships, people with epilepsy have an additional burden. When do I share the fact that I have epilepsy?

One of my patients, Andrea (not her real name), age 32, who mostly has simple partial and complex partial seizures shared her experience with this issue. You will see that her story is somewhat specific to her situation and seizure types. The fact that her seizures are *relatively* milder influences her approach. If she were having frequent, convulsive seizures, there would be different safety issues and earlier disclosure of the diagnosis might be important.

> When meeting someone new, I always find myself on the fence with the decision, "Do I tell this person I have epilepsy?" It's a tough decision to make. I will try to determine if I've had increased seizure activity recently, how often I will be around this person, and how I think they will take the information. In one instance, it has proven to be beneficial to inform someone in the early stages of a relationship.
>
> *(Continued)*

(*Continued*)

    I told my current partner shortly after meeting him, partly because I had been experiencing an increase in seizure activity. I explained that I have epilepsy, what happens during my seizures, and what he should do. Nothing more, nothing less; just the facts. On our third date, while at brunch, I felt my aura come on and blurted out loud, "I'm going to have a seizure." This is a typical pattern for me. It's not meant to alert anyone, the words just come out of my mouth. My partner said "OK," grabbed a phone so he could time the length of the seizure (as I had mentioned was helpful), and went back to eating while glancing up at me to make sure everything was proceeding as I explained it likely would. When I "came out" of my seizure—I didn't fall down and was just a little fuzzy with my thinking—he asked, "Was that it? Is it over?"

    "Yeah, that is pretty much it," I replied.

    "That's not a big deal at all!" he said. "It wasn't so bad. Are you feeling OK?"

    It took a moment to process the question because I was still somewhat recovering and also because I was floored at the nonchalant reaction—not because I was upset he was not more involved or sympathetic to the situation, but because he treated me as if it was no different than my having a headache or just having stubbed my toe. It was a relief. Often when telling people I have epilepsy they become afraid, treat me as if I were made of porcelain, or become so apologetic and devastated, as if I've told them I had a terminal illness. These reactions can give me a feeling of isolation. They can fuel the negativity I am already feeling about having a condition I have no control over. I had finally found someone that acknowledged me for . . . well, me, not my condition.

The issues to consider when deciding to tell others about one's epilepsy may be very different for someone with well-controlled seizures than someone with poorly controlled epilepsy. A balance has to be found between dependence (including support and its positive aspects) and independence. Friends, family members, and spouses often have a desire to be protective, especially if seizures are poorly controlled. This can provide a very effective line of defense against injury and harm. It can also change the focus of the relationship toward a more caregiving role. Changes in seizure control—including positive changes—can be disruptive and bring about unexpected changes. For example, becoming seizure free after epilepsy surgery would seem to be purely a cause for celebration. But it can bring with it what some have called a "burden of wellness." There may be more demands and expectations regarding school or work and unrealistic expectations for sudden reversals in longstanding disability. The caregiver aspect of relationships may become less important or no longer needed.

Ultimately, sharing the diagnosis of epilepsy with someone close to you can be an important step. Like all sharing in relationships, it may make you feel vulnerable, but it is also an opportunity to grow closer and develop shared goals.

When seizures and epilepsy become stressors in a relationship, several options can be considered. Couples' counseling may help to reexamine negative patterns that have developed in the relationship surrounding (or unrelated to) epilepsy. Support groups can also be a useful outlet, as others with epilepsy have undoubtedly had some of the same challenges. And finally, education efforts that reduce the stigma of epilepsy can help to bring down unnecessary barriers.

Related Brain Conditions: Cognitive Problems and Psychological Issues

Cognitive (Thinking) Issues That Commonly Accompany Epilepsy

When people with epilepsy are asked about their greatest concerns, challenges with thinking and memory are consistently near the top of the list. In fact, some part of cognition, or thinking, is commonly affected in epilepsy. Because epilepsy is a brain disease, both the epilepsy and the cognitive issues often share common roots. Cognitive issues may even precede the development of epilepsy in some cases.

If you have noticed problems with thinking or memory, there may be several possible causes. Seizures themselves can temporarily interrupt normal thought processes, but the brain mostly "resets" itself between seizures. However, if epilepsy is poorly controlled, and repeated seizures continue over many years, some people may experience progressive problems with thinking. Even single seizures, if unusually prolonged (status epilepticus), can sometimes worsen cognition. The underlying cause of the epilepsy might affect the normal function of that brain region. AEDs, which act on the brain, can potentially contribute to problems with thinking and cognition. And finally, psychological and psychiatric issues associated with epilepsy, including depression and anxiety, can have a strong influence on thinking ability and perceptions of cognitive deficits.

Elsa, aged 31, had experienced three secondarily generalized tonic-clonic seizures in her lifetime, all when she was 26 years old. Her neurological examination and EEG were normal, and her MRI scan of the brain did not identify a cause for the seizures. She quickly became seizure free on extended-release carbamazepine and required only infrequent visits with her doctor. She had mentioned some cognitive concerns in passing at previous clinic visits, but at a recent visit expressed this as a central concern. She worked as a technician in a research laboratory, and her supervisor had recently met with Elsa to review some errors she had made in following lab protocol. The errors had resulted in a failed experiment that had to be repeated. Her supervisor had not threatened her job, but Elsa was still concerned that it might be at risk if she made any more errors.

(Continued)

(*Continued*)

Elsa's doctor assessed the situation. She reviewed Elsa's testing and did some simple cognitive assessments in the clinic, which were normal. There was no evidence of problems with seizure control. A repeat MRI still showed no abnormalities.

Elsa was concerned that her AED might be responsible. A change in therapy was considered, but before this, her doctor referred her for neuropsychological testing.

Cognitive concerns are very common in people with epilepsy. In this case, Elsa had come to her doctor with concerns. However, there is some evidence that cognitive problems may be underreported. Some cognitive issues are present in well over half of people with epilepsy, and up to one-fourth may have an identifiable learning disability, but the range is large and overlaps with the normal and above average range. Some people with cognitive problems may be unaware of them, and for the doctor to simply ask about cognitive concerns may not be enough.

Among the various possible cognitive issues, problems with memory are the most commonly reported. This may especially be the case in people with temporal lobe epilepsy, which involves areas of the brain important for short-term memory, and in people who have had epilepsy for many years. Other common problems are slowing in processing speed or reaction time, trouble with maintaining attention, and difficulty with **executive function**. "Executive function" refers to planning and higher-level decision making. This level of thinking often involves holding several different ideas or possibilities in mind at the same time and having the mental flexibility to weigh options, see patterns, and make good choices.

What can be done to address cognitive concerns in people with epilepsy? First, problems need to be identified. As just suggested, this may require some inquiry and testing by the doctor. Sometimes more detailed testing by a neuropsychologist can be very helpful in defining areas of difficulty.

If the cognitive difficulty is in part related to the underlying cause of the epilepsy (for example, a traumatic brain injury from years ago), there may be limited direct treatment to address it. However, there are other important contributing issues to consider.

For instance, if seizures are poorly controlled, every effort should be made to improve control. The effect of seizures over many years on cognition is still incompletely understood. However, there is concern that, for at least some people with poorly controlled seizures over many years, a progressive decline in cognitive ability may occur. Some studies in people with poorly controlled seizures have shown faster loss of brain tissue than would be expected with normal aging.

At the same time, the risk of AED therapy contributing to cognitive problems must be considered. Responses to different AEDs vary widely, and these responses are somewhat individual. However, some medications (for example, phenobarbital and topiramate) are especially prone to causing cognitive problems. Some of the newer AEDs are less likely to contribute to cognitive problems. Often **polytherapy** (treatment with more than one AED) is more problematic than **monotherapy** (single drug therapy). If they cause cognitive problems, AEDs are most likely to affect processing speed, attention, and the ability to multitask, although memory and verbal skills may also be affected.

Finally, mood problems, specifically depression, can have a major influence. Depression can especially affect an individual's *perception* of their cognitive abilities or deficits. When an individual self-reports cognitive problems, there is often a close connection with mood and depression and often a looser connection with actual performance on cognitive tests.

Elsa returned from the neuropsychologist to see her doctor. The testing showed that most of her cognitive abilities fell in the average range. The neuropsychologist identified a number of stressors at home, as well as signs of mild to moderate depression. Elsa's doctor arranged for counseling to address the issues of concern in her home and initiated depression treatment. She also recognized that Elsa's average test scores might represent a decline from her previous performance— she had been a straight-A student all through school. If her cognitive concerns remained after treatment of depression and addressing her numerous stressors, they agreed to look at possible changes in AED therapy.

AEDs may often feel like the most visible cause of cognitive concerns. But before attributing all cognitive problems to AED therapy, it is worth considering other common contributors: the underlying cause of the epilepsy, the effect of recurrent seizures, and the sometimes hidden but powerful effects of mood and depression.

Psychiatric Issues That Commonly Accompany Epilepsy

Psychiatric problems are much more common in people with epilepsy than in those without seizures, adding to the already substantial burden of managing epilepsy. More than one-third of people with epilepsy will deal with psychiatric issues in the course of their epilepsy. While social stresses of having epilepsy may contribute, this is often a minor factor. More often, psychiatric disorders in epilepsy are the result of one or more of the following biological factors:

- The underlying cause of the epilepsy has disturbed brain function in areas that regulate mood and behavior

- The effect of intermittent seizures
- The effect of AED therapy

Thus much of the increase in mood and anxiety problems in people with epilepsy is a direct result of changes in brain chemistry. Entire books can and have been written on psychiatric issues associated with epilepsy. Here we will focus on three important areas: depression, anxiety, and psychosis.

Depression

The relationship between epilepsy and depression is complex. As previously mentioned, much of the depression seen in people with epilepsy is the result of biochemical changes in the brain. But it is not as simple as epilepsy or its treatments causing depression. There is also a connection in the reverse direction. That is to say, people who have depression are also more likely to develop epilepsy than the general population. This certainly strengthens the idea of a biological link between the brain systems involved in epilepsy and those that produce depression.

If you have depression, you may have noticed it has some relationship to your seizures. Some people will notice a change in mood as a sign of an impending seizure. One of my patients becomes withdrawn, depressed, and fearful, and knows that this is a sign that her seizures are about to begin. She often will have a cluster of seizures over 2 to 3 days, and then not have any further seizures for a month or more. It is also not unusual for mood changes to temporarily follow seizures. Another one of my patients had his major seizures controlled with AED therapy, but he continued having intermittent auras (simple partial seizures). These were brief events lasting 15 to 30 seconds without any change in his level of alertness. The worst and most disabling aspect of his auras was the mood changes that followed the brief auras. He typically felt intensely depressed for several hours or up to half a day after, and was able to function in only a limited way on days that he had auras.

For many people, however, this timed relationship between seizures and depression may not be seen. Most common is what is termed "interictal depression"—depression that is present in between seizures, or without a timed relationship to them. This can look exactly like depression in someone without epilepsy.

Some AEDs can bring on or worsen depression, as will be discussed in Chapter 10. Those that increase brain inhibition by boosting the brain chemical GABA are often included in this group, including phenobarbital, benzodiazepine medications (for example, clonazepam and diazepam), tiagabine, and vigabatrin. Other AEDs more commonly associated with depression include levetiracetam, topiramate, zonisamide, felbamate, and perampanel. Mood changes with AEDs can be somewhat unpredictable, however, and any possible relationship with starting or changing doses of an AED should be investigated.

When depression accompanies epilepsy, the important thing to know is that depression in epilepsy is treatable. Neurologists or primary care providers may decide to treat depression, or they may refer people with epilepsy to a mental health specialist such as a psychiatrist or psychiatric nurse practitioner. There are a few basic principles that they will follow. Medical treatment usually begins with a medication in the class called selective serotonin reuptake inhibitors (SSRIs), which are generally safe and effective for treating depression in people with epilepsy (for example, fluoxetine, sertraline, or citalopram). A related group of antidepressants called serotonin-norepinephrine reuptake inhibitors (SNRIs) are also often good choices (for example, venlafaxine). Older antidepressants called tricyclic antidepressants (TCAs) can be used, but since they are more likely to cause side effects and can occasionally worsen seizures, they are less preferred. The antidepressant bupropion (Wellbutrin) should generally be avoided, as it can increase seizures, especially at high doses.

When prescribing an antidepressant, doctors will try to avoid possible interactions with AEDs. Some of the AEDs, especially older enzyme-inducing AEDs, can make antidepressants less effective when given at typical doses. Some of the antidepressants can also affect levels of certain of the AEDs. If your depression seemed to appear or worsen after starting a new AED, you should make your doctor aware, and that treatment should be reconsidered.

The importance of identifying and treating depression in epilepsy cannot be overemphasized. As will be discussed in Chapter 10, a higher rate of suicidal thoughts and behaviors occur in people with epilepsy; diagnosis and treatment of depression can minimize this risk. Just as important, quality of life is strongly tied to depression and mood. In fact, a much stronger connection exists between *mood* and quality of life than between *number of seizures* and quality of life.

Anxiety

Anxiety is the second most common psychiatric disorder seen in people with epilepsy. Anxiety affects somewhere between one-sixth and one-fourth of people with epilepsy. There are different types of anxiety disorders, including generalized anxiety, panic disorder, obsessive-compulsive disorder (OCD), and posttraumatic stress disorder (PTSD).

Not infrequently, symptoms of anxiety can present diagnostic challenges.

Jackie was 31 when she started having episodes of intense fear and anxiety. These seemed to come on in normal, relaxed settings, without any trigger. Sometimes they woke her up out of sleep. Each episode lasted only about 30 seconds and then resolved, leaving her feeling tired. Her primary care provider thought she was having panic attacks and started her on

(Continued)

(*Continued*)
medication for this, but it didn't help. Two months later, she experienced her first generalized tonic-clonic seizure, which was preceded by the same exact feeling of intense anxiety and fear. In retrospect, she had been having simple partial seizures, not panic attacks, all along.

Some brain areas involved in temporal and frontal lobe seizures are tied to emotional centers in the brain that regulate fear and anxiety. Thus a simple partial seizure arising from those areas can produce symptoms that can often be mistaken for a panic attack. To make diagnosis even more difficult, someone in the midst of a panic attack may seem quite detached from his or her environment, suggesting a possible incorrect diagnosis of seizures. Anxiety symptoms that directly result from seizures usually differ from psychologically based panic attacks in several ways (see Box 3–1).

BOX 3-1 Features More Suggestive of Seizures Than Panic Attacks

- Seizures are usually brief (seizures typically last for 30–60 seconds; panic attacks may commonly last for 10 minutes or more)
- Seizures are stereotyped—they follow the same sequence of events each time; panic attacks may be more variable
- Seizures are not generally triggered by a specific situation (they come "out of the blue"); some panic attacks are triggered by specific situations or circumstances
- Seizures may have other features, such as automatisms or confusion; panic attacks rarely involve confusion

Of course, if a panic attack leads directly into a bigger seizure, the diagnosis often becomes clear: The link has been established and the "panic attack" was actually the beginning of the seizure.

If you have seizures that produce anxiety symptoms, the most effective approach is getting better control of the seizures. If anxiety is a separate problem from your seizures, it still needs attention. Your doctor may use some of the same medications mentioned for depression—the SSRIs and, sometimes, the SNRIs. Benzodiazepine medications such as clonazepam are sometimes used in the short term. As long-term therapy, benzodiazepines have potential disadvantages of causing sleepiness, tolerance (the body gets used to the medication and the effect may wear off), and problems of withdrawal (worse anxiety and possibly seizures) if the dose is reduced or discontinued. Counseling or "talk therapy" may also be very helpful.

Psychosis

Psychosis is a state of disordered thinking. It involves a loss of contact with reality and is often accompanied by hallucinations (seeing or especially hearing things that are not really there). The best-known illness where psychosis is a major feature is schizophrenia. Psychosis is less common in epilepsy than depression and anxiety. Episodes of psychosis may be seen in a little over 5 percent of people with epilepsy.

Psychosis may appear before, after, or in between seizures, but the best-known and best-studied relationship is with **postictal psychosis**. Postictal psychosis means symptoms of psychosis that emerge after a seizure, or after a cluster of seizures, and then go away after a period of days or sometimes weeks.

In postictal psychosis, a typical sequence of events is often seen. Following what is often a more severe than usual seizure or cluster of seizures, there may be a delay of 24 to 48 hours before symptoms appear. During this time the only change may be decreased sleep (insomnia). Then symptoms may emerge that can look very much like schizophrenia. The sense of reality is disrupted, and thinking is disordered. People with postictal psychosis may be suspicious of the intentions of others (paranoid). Hearing voices that are not there is common.

Friends or family members who see these changes should know that emergency medical care is often needed. Short-term treatment selected from a group of medicines called antipsychotic medications is often very effective. The treating doctor will know that older antipsychotic medications are more likely to cause side effects and that some can worsen seizures; therefore, he or she will be more likely to use the newer antipsychotic medications, often called atypical antipsychotics. Among these, only one—clozapine—should be avoided because of the potential risk of worsening seizures.

Some people are prone to repeat episodes of postictal psychosis. If you are in this situation, preventive treatment is often used. When you start to show the early signs of impending postictal psychosis (usually insomnia following a seizure or seizures), it is often possible to take a short course of an atypical antipsychotic medication at home to avoid the development of psychosis and the need for emergency care.

Some AEDs can produce or contribute to symptoms of psychosis. If you are taking phenobarbital, topiramate, levetiracetam, or others, your doctor may consider whether a change from these medications might help. However, it is important to make changes carefully and only under your doctor's supervision. Abrupt withdrawal from medications has also been reported to produce psychosis.

Sometimes treatment for postictal psychosis is delayed or avoided out of fear that antipsychotic medications could worsen seizures. If the preceding principles are followed, the risk of increased seizures is small and usually overshadowed by the benefits of treating the psychosis.

Sudden Unexpected Death in Epilepsy

It has been known for years, and better understood recently, that people with epilepsy have higher rates of sudden death than those who do not have epilepsy. The condition of **sudden unexpected death in epilepsy (SUDEP)** received a lot of publicity in 1998 when Olympic star Florence Griffith Joyner ("Flo Jo") died at the age of 38 from a nighttime seizure. Her death was attributed to SUDEP.

SUDEP can be a frightening thing to consider, and this is one reason why it is not discussed as often as it should be. A doctor or nurse might think, "Why should I scare my patient?" or "The risk of sudden death is higher in people with epilepsy, but still pretty small; what good would it do?" In fact, there are several important reasons to talk about and become educated about SUDEP. But let's start at the beginning.

SUDEP is defined as a sudden unexpected death in someone who has epilepsy, with some important limits. Although the risk of death from injury or drowning is also somewhat higher in people with epilepsy, these are not considered SUDEP. Death from an unusually prolonged seizure (status epilepticus) is also excluded from the SUDEP definition. In SUDEP, there is often evidence of a recent seizure, and no other cause of death is apparent.

Why Does SUDEP Occur?

This is being intensively studied, but the answers are still incomplete. A number of different factors may come together to produce SUDEP. Certain people may be at higher risk on a genetic basis, but there is no gene test to see who is at greatest risk for SUDEP. Seizures may rarely cause heart rhythm disturbances. Having a fast heartbeat during a seizure is very common and generally not cause for alarm. But rarely, a seizure can cause the heart rate to slow, or even stop briefly, and this may contribute to SUDEP. When SUDEP or near-SUDEP has been witnessed, breathing difficulties have often been reported. Following a severe seizure, there may, rarely, be a decreased drive to breathe. People who suffer SUDEP (like in sudden infant death syndrome, or SIDS) are often lying face down, and the decreased drive to breathe, the decreased responsiveness after a seizure, and partial blockage of the airway from lying face down may all contribute. Likely a number of these factors may combine in a "perfect storm" that produces SUDEP.

Just How Common Is SUDEP?

Taking everyone with epilepsy together, the frequency of SUDEP is about 1 for every 1,000 person-years. That number is a little hard to attach a meaning to. For comparison, let's look at the risk of sudden cardiac death in otherwise healthy young adults. For example, we hear every so often in the press about a young athlete who has suffered sudden cardiac death on the playing field. Though well publicized, the risk in that setting is about 1 for every 50,000 person-years, or about 50 times less than the risk of SUDEP in someone with epilepsy. So SUDEP is a serious risk and worth learning about.

Not all people with epilepsy are at equal risk for SUDEP. People at the highest risk for SUDEP include the following:

- Those with a history of generalized tonic-clonic seizures, especially frequent GTCs
- Those taking many AEDs
- Those with subtherapeutic (too low to be protective) AED levels
- Those undergoing frequent AED changes
- Young adults
- Those with early-onset epilepsy who have had seizures for many years

Among these, having severe epilepsy with frequent generalized tonic-clonic seizures, especially at night during sleep, is probably the strongest risk factor. Some other risk factors on the list, such as taking many AEDs, probably just identify those with more severe epilepsy; the medications themselves don't seem to put people at risk.

As noted, some doctors are reluctant to talk to their patients about SUDEP. Sometimes this might just be because it is an uncomfortable topic to discuss. At other times, they may not want to make patients who may already be suffering from anxiety more anxious. Some argue that telling people about SUDEP denies their right to *not* know (sort of an "ignorance is bliss" argument).

On the other side of the scale, there are many strong reasons to discuss SUDEP, at some point, with many or most people with epilepsy. It follows the basic principle of telling the truth. Even if it makes people anxious, it still allows for a discussion and expression of that anxiety. Many people may already have read or heard about SUDEP and might be even more anxious than they need to be. Parents or family members of someone who dies of SUDEP may be hurt and angry that this tragic event that happened to their loved one was not even discussed as a possibility. But perhaps the strongest reason to discuss SUDEP is that some measures can be taken to reduce its risk.

What Can Be Done to Reduce the Risk of SUDEP?

Some of the risk factors, like age and seizure type, can't be modified. However, regular medication dosing can make a difference. One very important study looked at people who were frequently irregular in dosing their AEDs. They found that these people were at about a three times higher risk of an epilepsy-related death than those who took their medications regularly. *That* can be modified. If you have been taking AEDs for a long period of time, it is easy to develop a false sense of security or feeling of complacency: "I'm not sure my AEDs are doing much," or "Maybe I don't really need my AEDs." This study should remind everyone that any changes with AEDs need to be done very cautiously and only under expert guidance.

There is much more that we need to learn about how to prevent SUDEP beyond simply taking AEDs regularly. Many cases of SUDEP happen with nighttime seizures. Having a bed partner who can respond to a seizure appears to be somewhat protective. Probably having someone to reposition and help awaken someone after seizures may be protective. If you don't have a bed partner, some other means of nighttime supervision may be important if you are at high risk. For some people, this could be regular nighttime checks by family members or group home staff. New technology is rapidly developing that may help with seizure detection and alerts to family members or caregivers. CPR training for family and friends of those with severe epilepsy is advisable. Continuing to pursue better seizure control is also very important, including considering epilepsy surgery if you have medically refractory epilepsy. People with medically refractory epilepsy are at high risk for SUDEP, and evidence from some studies suggests that successful epilepsy surgery can substantially reduce the risk of SUDEP.

Recently, a partnership between scientists, doctors, patients, families, and other interested parties has been formed to advance the understanding and prevention of SUDEP. Efforts by groups such as this one, called Partners Against Mortality in Epilepsy (PAME; pame. aesnet.org) will lead to the next advances in SUDEP prevention.

Making Clinic Visits Successful

A few small steps can go a long way toward making your first visit with the neurologist successful (see Box 3–2):

- Be prepared and organized
- Bring a friend or family member
- Prioritize

BOX 3-2 A Visit with the Neurologist

Check-in: A check-in procedure, including registration in the medical record system and a check of your vital signs (weight, blood pressure, pulse)

History: A review of medical history by the neurologist with a focus on the symptoms that prompted the visit

Examination: This often includes some general medical examination (for example, listening to the heart and lungs), but focuses on the neurological examination, in which the neurologist may examine:

- Thinking and memory using a series of questions
- The head and neck, including eye movements
- Muscles and strength
- Sensation
- Reflexes (tapping with a reflex hammer)
- Coordination
- Walking and balance

Discussion: Neurologists should provide a summary of what they think is going on. They will discuss whether any other testing is needed to establish a diagnosis. They will discuss whether treatment is needed, and if so, what treatment is recommended. Often some decisions need to be made, and the neurologist may involve you in this decision-making process. There should be some time at the end of the visit for questions.

Be Prepared and Organized

You will have a limited amount of time to see your neurologist, and you don't want to use all of that time trying to locate information.

The first step is to check in. You may find the visit less stressful if you arrive with extra time to spare (approximately 30 minutes) to make sure that check-in is completed before your scheduled appointment time. Bring insurance information and ID cards with you.

If you have been evaluated previously, including in an emergency department, try to obtain those records, including copies of any brain scans, in advance of your visit and bring these with you. Most hospital and health care facilities will provide these for you on request. It is also a good idea to keep a copy for your own records. Complete any forms the clinic has sent you in advance of the visit. Take a few minutes to organize your health story also. Your neurologist is likely to ask you about the following areas, so being prepared, including making lists of the following items in advance, will make this process more efficient:

- Describe briefly your episodes or possible seizures (why you are there)
- List other medical conditions and surgeries that you have had
- List any medications you take
- List any medication allergies (bad reactions to medications) that you have experienced
- Have a short list of any conditions that run in the family—especially any seizures or brain diseases
- Be prepared to answer questions honestly about tobacco, alcohol, and illicit drug use. It doesn't help anyone if you are not truthful about substance use

If you are an established patient and are coming for return visits, one of the most important things you can do is to be prepared and organized with information about seizures that have occurred during the interval since your last visit. This means keeping a seizure calendar or diary. This does not have to be elaborate. My patients have taken a number of different approaches depending on their time and level of computer skills. Here are some ideas for different types of seizure calendars or diaries:

1. *Paper seizure calendar* (Figure 3–1). This is a very effective approach. A simple sheet of paper or a pocket calendar with the dates and times of seizures marked is incredibly helpful in understanding whether a change in treatment has been successful. Enhancing the simple calendar with brief descriptions of symptoms or possible triggers can be useful.

2. *Electronic spreadsheet.* Some people prefer to track their seizures electronically. Sometimes they will record notes on paper and then transfer them to the computer. One advantage of this approach is that the notes are typed and easily readable by the provider. Many people also like that they are able to keep an ongoing record of their seizure control over time in the stored electronic record.

3. *Internet/Web-based approaches.* For those more digitally inclined, there are a number of options for tracking seizures using secure Internet-based approaches. One of the best options is "My Epilepsy Diary" at epilepsy.com. In addition to the above advantages, it has smartphone apps to allow recording of events wherever you are, and it can also track medications and graph the results.

Whatever approach you choose, the principle is the same. Good decisions are based on good information.

Bring a Friend or Family Member

Having a friend or family member with you at the visit can be helpful in several ways.

A friend or family member, especially one who has witnessed your seizures, may be able to provide valuable information. If you have experienced an event or seizure that involved loss or alteration of consciousness, it will be hard for you to describe everything that happened in the course of the event. It will be very helpful for your doctor to talk to both you and someone who has witnessed your

SEIZURE CALENDAR

Seizure Calendar for: _____ **Dates:** _____ **to** _____ **Year** _____

Seizure Key: (Describe type of seizures and label by letter, using 1 letter for each different type of seizure. Record number of seizures using seizure key on the dates they occur. Females can note the day of their menstrual cycle next to 'cycle' day. Note if any triggers such as missed or changes in meds, change in sleep, diet or activity; stress; other illness.)

Type A: _____ **Type C:** _____

Type B: _____ **Type D:** _____

SUNDAY	MONDAY	TUESDAY	WEDNESDAY	THURSDAY	FRIDAY	SATURDAY
Date: Cycle: Event:	Date: Cycle: Event:	Date: Cycle: Event:	Date: Cycle: Event:	Date: Cycle: Event:	Date: Cycle: Event:	Date: Cycle: Event:
Date: Cycle: Event:	Date: Cycle: Event:	Date: Cycle: Event:	Date: Cycle: Event:	Date: Cycle: Event:	Date: Cycle: Event:	Date: Cycle: Event:
Date: Cycle: Event:	Date: Cycle: Event:	Date: Cycle: Event:	Date: Cycle: Event:	Date: Cycle: Event:	Date: Cycle: Event:	Date: Cycle: Event:
Date: Cycle: Event:	Date: Cycle: Event:	Date: Cycle: Event:	Date: Cycle: Event:	Date: Cycle: Event:	Date: Cycle: Event:	Date: Cycle: Event:
Date: Cycle: Event:	Date: Cycle: Event:	Date: Cycle: Event:	Date: Cycle: Event:	Date: Cycle: Event:	Date: Cycle: Event:	Date: Cycle: Event:

A service of the Epilepsy Foundation

FIGURE 3–1 Example of a seizure calendar.

events. If this is not possible, second best is to have any available witnesses write a short paragraph about what they observed. What did they first notice? What happened next? When did it end? What was the recovery period like? Sometimes an observer can contribute a key piece of information that helps to make the diagnosis.

I recently saw a man who had experienced rare "spells." From his description, it was very hard to tell what was going on. His wife had witnessed one, and when I brought her in from the waiting room (with his permission), it was incredibly helpful. She was able to clearly describe lip-smacking automatisms and a period of marked confusion after the spell. The working diagnosis quickly changed from "unknown" to "likely complex partial seizure," a diagnosis later confirmed by EEG.

A lot of information can come from your first visit to the neurologist. Another role for a friend or family member is as a note taker. Things may make sense in the moment, but it is very helpful to have notes to refer to after the visit, when some of the details may have been forgotten.

Finally, a visit to the neurologist for the first time can be stressful! A friend or family member can be a good source of support as you are trying to understand how and why things are changing and how to manage new realities.

Prioritize

There may not be time at your first visit to the neurologist to answer *every* question that you might have. That is okay, as long as you take a little time in advance to prioritize. I recommend writing out a short list of the two or three top concerns or questions that you don't want to leave this visit without asking. Consider telling your neurologist about them at the *start* of the visit, so that he or she can plan time at the end to address them and be thinking about them during the course of the visit.

A Few Final Tips

- Be positive. A friendly approach, cooperation, courtesy, and respect will go a long way toward building a positive relationship with your doctor and team. This will definitely pay off over the years!
- If communication is not working well despite your best efforts, consider the options for changing to another provider.
- Advocate for yourself! Your doctor will guide you, but it is ultimately your health that is being discussed—don't completely hand this important issue off to someone else!
- Make sure you are clear on all instructions before leaving the clinic. Ask questions if things are unclear.
- Make sure there is an understanding about how issues will be handled between clinic visits. Do you know who to call if there are urgent concerns at night or on weekends?
- Keep telephone or electronic communications between clinic visits focused and brief. If there are complex issues to be discussed, try to schedule a clinic visit to discuss them.
- Be open to sharing information. A productive clinic visit requires a high level of trust. Your doctor may ask about sensitive topics. These may include drug and alcohol use, sexual function, family planning, and driving. The more you can be honest and straightforward in your answers, the better the care the doctor can provide.
- Educate yourself. You are reading this book, so you are already ahead of the game! You can be the best advocate for yourself and ask the best questions in clinic if you are well informed. This book may just be a starting point. The references in this book, as well as the resources of the Epilepsy Foundation and other advocacy groups, can help you meet this goal.

Chapter 4

How and Why Do Seizures Occur?

Basic Science of Epilepsy

Epilepsy experts and neuroscientists continue to puzzle over some of the most basic issues about epilepsy.

- What starts a seizure?
- Why does a seizure happen at a particular point in time?
- What allows a seizure to end?
- What changes can turn someone's brain from a not-likely-to-have-a-seizure brain into the condition of epilepsy—an "enduring predisposition to have seizures" as we learned in Chapter 2?

Sometimes the answers to the simple questions are the hardest to find. While great strides have been made in answering these questions, much work still remains. The goal of this chapter is to explain some basics about how seizures work and why this knowledge is important. Here we will discuss what is known about the mechanisms by which seizures arise. We will learn about the most common underlying *causes* of epilepsy in the next chapter.

Anyone can have a seizure. Under most circumstances, there is balance in the brain systems or "networks." Communication occurs across established pathways via tiny chemical and electrical signals. You might imagine that each of these signals is like an instrument in an orchestra. Each instrument has to play the right note at the right tempo and loudness to make a harmonious piece of music.

Together, these signals carry out all of the important work of the brain, from controlling movement, to allowing you to interpret the words on the page, and then later remember some of them and be able to tell a friend.

Balance of Excitation and Inhibition

Some brain connections and chemical messengers work to make "excitatory" signals in the brain. These signals make the connected brain cells *more likely* to fire. This is not a bad thing, and under normal circumstances these excitatory signals control many normal brain functions including (or especially) memory function. These connections and chemical messengers are balanced by "inhibitory" ones. These signals "cool things off" and make the connected brain cells *less likely* to fire. Normal brain function (see Figure 4–1) depends on a balance between excitation and inhibition in the billions of neurons and trillions of connections between these brain cells.

In epilepsy, this balance is disrupted, and the imbalance leads to seizures. You can imagine that either too much excitation (see Figure 4–2) or too little inhibition (Figure 4–3) could tip the scales in favor of seizures. It is as if the trumpet section of the orchestra got excited and started playing very quickly and loudly. Then the neighbors—the percussion and woodwinds—decided to join in, too.

What systems underlie these imbalances in excitation and inhibition? As you can imagine, this discussion could get very technical,

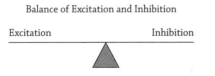

Balance of Excitation and Inhibition

Excitation   Inhibition

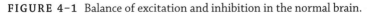

FIGURE 4-1 Balance of excitation and inhibition in the normal brain.

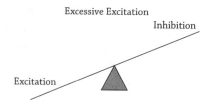

FIGURE 4-2 Imbalance of excitation and inhibition: too much excitation.

very quickly! We'll try to cover some of the basic systems in this chapter. Understanding how seizures work allows scientists to develop new treatments and may help you understand something about how the seizure medications to be discussed in Chapter 9 work. For any budding neuroscientists out there, we list some opportunities for further reading at the end of the book. For anyone less scientifically inclined, don't worry if you don't understand everything.

Epilepsy at the Level of the Brain Cell

Let's start with a single nerve cell, or **neuron**—the building block of the brain (Figure 4–4). Since brain function is all about communication between cells, how are these signals sent?

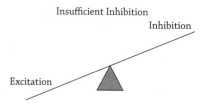

FIGURE 4-3 Imbalance of excitation and inhibition: too little inhibition.

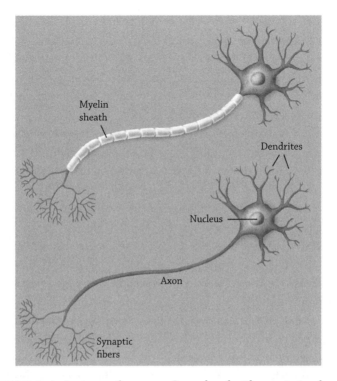

FIGURE 4-4 Anatomy of a neuron. Reproduced with permission from Caplan, L. *Navigating the Complexities of Stroke.*© American Academy of Neurology 2013. Adapted from http://pubs.niaaa.nih.gov/publications/arh25-3/175-184.htm.

Most neurons have several main parts:

- Cell body
- Dendrites
- Axon

In general, the cell body contains most of the machinery for the basic functions of the cell. The dendrites are specialized branches that receive signals from other neurons. The axon carries the main output from the neuron to its other connections.

Especially at these connection points between cells, the outer "skin" of the cell, or "cell membrane," contains channels or pores where particles can move in and out of the cell. These particles, or *ions*, like sodium, potassium, and chloride, carry an electrical charge. The ability of a neuron to send a signal depends on a balance of these ions inside and outside of the cell.

Some channels permit ions to move fairly freely in and out of the cell. Others have gates that regulate the flow of ions in and out of the cell. One of the most important gated channels is the sodium channel. When sodium channels open, the electrical charge of the cell is changed. When enough sodium channels open it can trigger an "action potential"—a strong electrical signal that is sent down the axon to neighboring cells to which they are connected. Sodium channels can open in response to chemical or electrical signals from other cells. The brain chemicals involved in this process are called **neurotransmitters**. Some neurotransmitters make a cell more likely to fire an electrical signal. These are called **excitatory neurotransmitters**. Others make a cell less likely to fire and are termed **inhibitory neurotransmitters**.

So far we have been discussing the signaling mechanisms of the normal brain. Even a normal brain can have a seizure. In certain situations—for example, if the balance of sodium in the body is very disturbed—someone with a normal brain can be tipped over into having a seizure. However, in someone with epilepsy, seizures can occur even in the absence of a major disturbance in brain chemistry. Instead, there is something different about both the brain cells and their connections that makes it easier for the brain to have a seizure.

In someone with epilepsy, changes in the opening of channels may make certain neurons likely to fire more rapidly. This may in turn lead connected cells to fire more rapidly. Picture a group of people in a stadium doing the "wave"—standing up when their neighbor stands up and causing a wave of movement across the stadium—and you have an idea how a seizure might spread across the brain. Cells in a seizure are firing more rapidly than usual and also more synchronously—together with their neighbors. In this way a seizure hijacks the normal mechanisms of brain communication, causing an "electrical storm" in the brain that interrupts normal communication. Surprisingly, it is not simple to explain why a seizure stops after a few seconds or minutes. The stop signal may be the result of both a release of inhibitory neurotransmitters and metabolic and energetic exhaustion of the cells involved in the seizure. When the seizure stops, the brain mostly "resets" and gradually recovers to the pre-seizure state.

Many of the medications used to treat epilepsy target these features we have been learning about. For example, some of the most commonly used antiepileptic medications act by blocking sodium channels in neurons. This makes them less likely to fire action potentials and therefore makes them less excitable (and less likely to cause seizures). Others may block excitatory neurotransmitters or boost inhibitory ones.

Epilepsy at the Network Level

The brain is highly interconnected and always changing (Figure 4–5).

Scientists call connected groups of neurons **networks**. While we once thought that we had a fixed number of brain cells that were slowly lost with aging, we now know that the situation is much more dynamic. Neurons are lost with aging, but new neurons are also born throughout adulthood. Even more, the connections between neurons—the **synapses**—are constantly changing. New connections are made. Old, unused connections are pruned away. The saying goes: "Cells that fire together, wire together." In other words, when certain pathways are used repeatedly, those connections are strengthened. This is the process that underlies the development of a new skill through practice. There is some evidence, at least in animals, that the brain may behave the same way in response to seizures. As more seizures occur, those pathways may

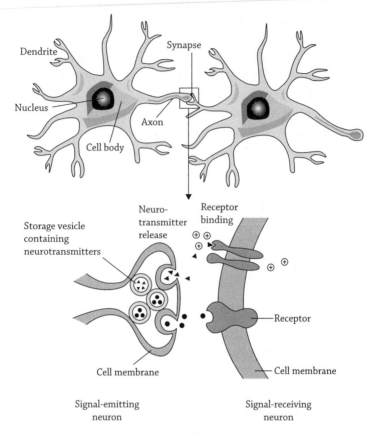

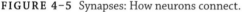

FIGURE 4-5 Synapses: How neurons connect.
Structural features of a typical nerve cell (i.e., neuron) and synapse. This
drawing shows the major components of a typical neuron, including the cell
body with the nucleus, the dendrites that receive signals from other neurons,
and the axon that relays nerve signals to others neurons at a specialized
structure called a synapse. When the nerve signal reaches the synapse, it
causes the release of chemical messengers (i.e., neurotransmitters) from
storage vesicles. The neurotransmitters travel across a minute gap between
the cells and then interact with protein molecules (i.e., receptors) located
in the membrane surrounding the signal-receiving neuron. This interaction
causes biochemical reactions that result in the generation, or prevention, of
a new nerve signal, depending on the type of neuron, neurotransmitter, and
receptor involved (Goodlett and Horn 2001).

be strengthened, and the brain may in effect become better at having seizures. It remains uncertain to what extent this process occurs in humans, but it is one of many reasons why doctors work with patients to get seizures controlled as quickly and as completely as possible. We don't currently have medications that help rewire the brain of someone with epilepsy so they are no longer prone to seizures. That is the ultimate goal—to use medications that not only suppress the symptoms (seizures) but that also treat the underlying epilepsy. Scientists worldwide are busy at work to solve this complex problem.

Don't worry too much about the technical details of this section. Here are the important takeaway points to keep in mind:

- Anyone can have a seizure.
- Seizures are caused by an imbalance between excitation and inhibition.
- People with epilepsy have some differences in their brains that makes the balance tip more easily toward excitation and seizures.
- Brain networks are complex, and changes that alter the balance of excitation and inhibition can develop over long periods of time.
- If we can understand the mechanisms, we can design treatments to correct the problem and prevent seizures.

A seizure can be a "final common path" for many different brain conditions that might even seem unrelated. In the next chapter, we'll explore some of these different specific causes of epilepsy, but as we do this, keep in mind that all of these causes in some way disturb the complex balance of excitation and inhibition.

Chapter 5

Who Develops Epilepsy?

In previous chapters I have emphasized that anyone can have a seizure. However, not everyone is equally likely to develop epilepsy. In this chapter, we will explore some of the most common causes of epilepsy. Causes of epilepsy are sometimes divided into those that are acquired—an event such as a traumatic brain injury that turns a previously normal brain into one with epilepsy—and genetic or inherited causes of epilepsy. Although this can be a useful way to think about the different causes of epilepsy, we will see that this division may be too simplistic.

While epilepsy can appear at any age, people in two age groups are most likely to develop epilepsy.

The first group is children. Many processes that affect the brain and lead to seizures first appear in childhood. These include genetic causes, abnormalities in the way the brain was formed (developmental malformations), problems with metabolism, and various injuries that may occur, including stroke (bleeding in the brain or blockage of blood flow to a part of the brain). A child's brain is very different from that of an adult. While much of brain development occurs before birth, many developmental processes continue in the first few years of life and beyond.

Since this book is focused on epilepsy in adolescents and adults, the many causes of epilepsy in children will not be discussed further here, but these basic ideas are important because many people first develop epilepsy in childhood that persists into adulthood. Some common causes of epilepsy in children are:

- Genetic conditions
- Brain injury from lack of oxygen around the time of birth
- Brain malformations
- Metabolic conditions
- Traumatic brain injury
- Brain infections (meningitis, encephalitis)
- Brain tumors
- Stroke (injury to the brain from lack of blood flow to or bleeding in part of the brain)

The second group is adults. Developing epilepsy in adulthood is also common; in fact, the largest group of people with new-onset epilepsy is adults over the age of 65. The causes in this age group are different than in children; some of the most common causes follow. As you can see, there is some overlap with the causes of epilepsy in children. However, by adulthood, most of the genetic and congenital causes have already appeared during childhood and are rarely the cause of new-onset seizures in adults. In people over age 65, the most common cause of new-onset epilepsy is stroke. Common causes of new-onset epilepsy in adults are:

- Stroke (injury to the brain from lack of blood flow to or bleeding in part of the brain)
- Traumatic brain injury
- Brain infection (meningitis, encephalitis)
- Neurodegenerative disease (Alzheimer's disease, multiple sclerosis)
- Brain tumor
- Blood vessel malformation
- Substance abuse

As we have seen, epilepsy can be a final common path resulting from many different brain abnormalities or injuries. The list is too long to discuss each of these exhaustively. We will look at some of the most common causes in the remainder of this chapter.

Genetic Causes of Epilepsy

Genetic abnormalities are a major cause of epilepsy. Epilepsy with a genetic cause means there is a problem with one or more genes. You may remember that humans have 23 pairs of chromosomes (one set from each parent), and our genes live on these chromosomes. In total, there are about 30,000 to 40,000 human genes. These genes contain the blueprints for human development, including brain development and function. When genes are copied, a certain amount of error occurs in the process. This process, called **mutation**, introduces changes into the genetic code for an individual. Many mutations do not cause any problems. Others can result in human disease, including epilepsy. In some cases, a mutation that causes epilepsy can be passed down through generations of a family (inherited). In other cases, the mutation may newly arise in an individual who has no family history of seizures or epilepsy.

How Do Genetic Problems Lead to Seizures?

Some genetic syndromes affect many body systems. For example, many people have heard of Down's syndrome, which affects many aspects of growth and development, including brain function. People with Down's syndrome are more likely to have seizures. But often the other problems associated with Down's syndrome take center stage. Seizures or epilepsy may be a minor or late feature of this condition. There are many genetic conditions like this in which seizures and epilepsy may be a small part of the larger disease or genetic syndrome. There are too many of these genetic syndromes that have epilepsy as one small part to discuss here. Instead, we will focus on conditions where epilepsy is the main or only feature of the genetic problem.

Many, but certainly not all, genetic causes of epilepsy first manifest with childhood seizures. However, other genetic causes of epilepsy may not appear until adolescence: the most common being juvenile myoclonic epilepsy, or JME, which was discussed in Chapter 2.

A range of genetic causes of epilepsy are known. The simplest and best understood are single-gene defects leading to epilepsy. In these conditions, a single gene is altered or missing, producing epilepsy. In Chapter 4, we learned a little about how seizures work and about the importance of the balance between excitation and inhibition in the brain. We learned that much of this balance is determined by ion channels that let substances such as sodium, potassium, and calcium in and out of the brain cells.

You might predict that if something was altered with these ion channels, it might make brain cells more likely to fire (more excitable) and lead to epilepsy. You would be right! In fact, many of the simple, single-gene defects that lead to epilepsy involve mutations in these ion channels. Although many of these single-gene defects have been identified, they make up only a tiny percentage of all cases of epilepsy—less than 1 percent. Still, the understanding of how changes in different channels can lead to epilepsy has given scientists great insight into the mechanisms by which seizures are produced and has led to the development of new medications for epilepsy.

This would seem to indicate that genetic causes of epilepsy are rare, but that is not the case. However, once we leave the single-gene defects, things get more complicated. Most genetic epilepsies are not the result of a problem with a single gene. Instead, small changes in several genes may add up to produce epilepsy. This makes it much harder to identify the genes involved in producing epilepsy in a given person. It also makes genetic testing much more difficult (see Chapter 7).

It has been estimated that around 30 percent of epilepsy may have a primarily genetic cause. Scientists have also recognized that the division of the causes of epilepsy into genetic and acquired (for example, acquired as the result of a head injury) is probably too simple. It is proposed that there may be seizure susceptibility genes that may determine who is at greatest risk for developing epilepsy following a brain injury. Let me give an example. Imagine that three people are walking under a construction site, and three bricks of equal size fall from the same height and strike each of these three people on the head in the same place, causing identical traumatic brain injuries. One of these people goes on to develop seizures and epilepsy as a result of the injury while the other two do not. Why would this be? Scientists speculate that a complex combination of genes determines someone's susceptibility to seizures. Some people might be genetically more prone to developing seizures and require only a minor brain injury to "tip them over" into epilepsy. Others may have genes that make the brain more resistant to developing epilepsy. As scientists' understanding of genetics continues to rapidly grow, we will also grow in our understanding of the complex contribution of genetics to epilepsy.

If you have epilepsy, you might worry about the risk that your children might also develop epilepsy. The experts in this area are in a specialized field called *medical genetics*. If this is a concern for you, you may want to consider talking with a genetic counselor about your specific situation. In general, because of the complex genetics in most forms of epilepsy, the risk is often not as great as you might think. Very few of the genetic epilepsies are ones in which a high percentage (for example, half or a quarter) of children inherit the condition. Overall, there is about a 2 to 4 times increased risk of epilepsy in close relatives of someone with known epilepsy. In most cases, this means a less than 10 percent risk of passing on the epilepsy, and the risk is probably much lower in situations where the parent has a clearly acquired cause of epilepsy, such as an infection or a stroke.

Currently, the ability to do specific testing to find a genetic cause for your epilepsy is very limited, but this will certainly change in the future. This topic is explored in more detail in Chapter 7.

Acquired Causes of Epilepsy

At the other end of the spectrum from those epilepsies with a primarily *genetic* cause are epilepsies with a primarily *acquired* cause. This means that something happens to the brain of someone who is not otherwise prone to seizures to convert it from a brain that is unlikely to have seizures to one with "an enduring predisposition to seizures."

> Nikki had never experienced seizures before the night she went out drinking with her friends, then got behind the wheel and drove her car at high speed off the road and into a tree. She sustained a serious brain injury, with damage to both of her frontal lobes, and was in a coma for 2 days. She returned home 60 days after the accident following extensive rehabilitation efforts. She was struggling with many issues, including headaches, trouble sleeping, poor memory, and other cognitive problems. About 9 months after the accident, her family noticed some periods of decreased responsiveness and mild confusion, but they chalked it up to fatigue. It wasn't until one of these confusional episodes preceded a generalized tonic-clonic seizure that the connection with epilepsy was made. The brain injury, and subsequent rewiring of brain circuits over the months that followed, led to her epilepsy. Those changes converted a normal brain to one that was now prone to spontaneous seizures. Nikki had an acquired epilepsy.

Remember that for many people, it may not be so simple, and there may be a complex mix of genetic and acquired factors that lead to the development of epilepsy. In most cases, these acquired brain problems produce focal-onset seizures—simple partial, complex partial, or secondarily generalized seizures, or a combination of these. What are some of those acquired causes?

Traumatic Brain Injury

Traumatic brain injury (TBI), as in Nikki's case, is a well-known cause of seizures. However, not all traumatic brain injuries create the same risk of epilepsy.

Often TBI is broken up into mild, moderate, and severe categories. Definitions vary, but often mild TBI describes a head injury with no loss of consciousness, or with loss of consciousness that lasts less than 30 minutes. While TBI of this type can cause many problems (for example, headache, dizziness, memory difficulty), it is not clearly associated with an increased risk of developing epilepsy. In the clinic, we routinely ask about traumatic brain injury, and I'm always amazed how nearly everyone has hit his head on the "monkey bars" or has been hit in the head by a baseball. Bumps to the head in toddlers learning to walk are common. As humans, we always try to make sense of things, and lacking another identified cause, it is tempting to blame the seizures on a minor TBI. But this kind of very mild TBI rarely causes epilepsy.

Moderate TBI (often defined as head injury with loss of consciousness greater than 30 minutes but less than 24 hours) is clearly associated with an increased risk of developing epilepsy. Severe TBI (loss of consciousness for more than 24 hours) places someone at relatively high risk for developing epilepsy, especially if there is an injury that penetrates the skull (for example, a bullet wound).

Epilepsy can develop shortly after a traumatic brain injury or sometimes years later, as the brain recovers, rewires, and creates more excitable circuits in the process. How long after a TBI can epilepsy develop? There is no absolute cutoff, and to some extent it depends on the context. If someone had a severe TBI, has no other risk factors for epilepsy, and begins having seizures 5 years later, it would seem likely that the epilepsy is related to the TBI, even though the TBI occurred years earlier. On the other hand, if someone had a mild TBI 10 years earlier and has an alternative explanation for the seizures (for example, a strong family history of seizures), it is much less likely that the TBI is the principal cause of the epilepsy.

Brain Tumors

Brain tumors commonly cause seizures. Both tumors that begin in the brain (called **primary brain tumors**) and tumors that begin in another part of the body, such as lung cancer or breast cancer, and spread to the brain (called **metastatic tumors**) can cause epilepsy. Tumors that are large and rapidly growing may first cause symptoms such as headaches, weakness, or other neurological difficulties before the seizures appear. Slow-growing tumors are more likely to appear with seizures as the initial symptom. In these people, a seizure may be the first clue that a brain tumor is present. As we will see in Chapter 7, everyone with new-onset seizures should have at least one good-quality brain magnetic resonance imaging (MRI) test. It is important to not miss some potential causes of epilepsy, such as brain tumors that might require additional treatment beyond the control of seizures.

Stroke

Stroke is the most common cause of new-onset epilepsy in people over the age of 65 years. Most people who have a stroke do not go on to develop epilepsy. In fact, fewer than 10 percent of those with stroke will develop epilepsy. But because strokes are so common, they are still a leading cause of epilepsy.

There are two main types of stroke. The first is called **ischemic stroke**. In an ischemic stroke, the flow of blood to part of the brain is blocked, resulting in permanent injury to that part of the brain. The second type is called a **hemorrhagic stroke**. In this type of stroke bleeding occurs within the brain or across the surface of the brain.

Both types of stroke can cause seizures, but not all strokes produce the same risk of epilepsy. Remember that seizures are generated in the cortex, the wrinkled outer surface of the brain where the brain cells live. Strokes that involve lower parts of the brain (the brainstem) or the wiring that connects different areas of cortex (the white matter) are much less likely to produce epilepsy.

Ischemic strokes involving the cortex do increase the risk of epilepsy, especially if the stroke is large.

Hemorrhagic strokes are most likely to result in new-onset epilepsy. The risk of developing epilepsy after a hemorrhagic stroke is about twice that from an ischemic stroke. The reason is likely that some of the breakdown products of blood, including forms of hemoglobin, are very toxic to the cortex. As the blood is reabsorbed after a hemorrhagic stroke, some of these blood products remain, acting as an irritant to the cortex and producing seizures.

Blood Vessel Malformations

Abnormalities of the blood vessels in the brain can lead to seizures. Some epilepsy results from abnormalities of veins in the brain, such as **cavernous hemangiomas**. A cavernous hemangioma is a clump of thin-walled veins in the brain that are fragile and prone to bleeding or leaking blood products into the surrounding brain. Other malformations consist of abnormal connections between the arteries and veins in the brain, called **arteriovenous malformations,** or **AVMs**. These AVMs can pose a high risk of serious bleeding and sometimes require surgical treatment. As with brain tumors, it is important to identify these malformations using brain imaging. Surgical treatment, if indicated, can often reduce both the risk of bleeding and seizures.

Malformations of Brain Development

Brain development is a highly complex process. The major brain structures of a baby develop early in pregnancy, and more subtle ongoing development happens throughout late pregnancy and for many years following birth. Sometimes this complex and elegant developmental process can be disturbed in major or minor ways. Major abnormalities of brain development are usually identified shortly after birth and may often cause intellectual disability (formerly called mental retardation), delayed development, and seizures. On the other hand, more subtle abnormalities of brain development may not become apparent for many years and can appear during teenage or adult years as new-onset seizures. As technology has improved and brain imaging tests such as MRI produce more and more detailed pictures of the brain, many people who previously had an "unknown" cause for epilepsy are now found to have small malformations of brain development. These small malformations often do not cause apparent problems with brain function, such as thinking or memory. However, they do affect the way the brain cells in that region are wired together, often leading to seizures. If seizures don't respond to medications, these small malformations can sometimes be safely removed surgically (Chapter 11).

Other Acquired Brain Abnormalities

The other possible acquired causes of epilepsy are too numerous to review in detail here but may commonly include brain infections (meningitis, encephalitis, brain abscess), various causes of brain inflammation, neurodegenerative diseases such as Alzheimer's disease, injury to the middle part of the temporal lobe called hippocampal sclerosis, and many others.

Unknown Causes of Epilepsy

Finally, a sizable group of people remain in whom the cause of epilepsy cannot be identified. This is a "good news, bad news" situation. First, the good news: In general, it can be reassuring to be told you are in this group, as it means none of the more concerning causes for epilepsy, such as a brain tumor, have been identified. The bad news? It is often frustrating to be told the cause is not known, because there is no answer to the question "Why do I have epilepsy?" As medical technology continues to improve, especially in the area of brain imaging and genetics, many previously unknown causes may be revealed.

This chapter emphasizes that epilepsy does not have a single cause. There are a host of genetic and acquired causes of epilepsy, and probably many that are a mix of the two. Despite all of the tools available for diagnosis, the underlying cause of epilepsy in many people remains unknown. The next chapter looks at some of the thought processes and tools used to establish a diagnosis of epilepsy.

Chapter 6

Establishing the Diagnosis of Epilepsy

Sometimes the diagnosis of epilepsy is obvious. If your epilepsy began with a series of generalized tonic-clonic or "grand mal" seizures that were witnessed, there may have been little doubt about the diagnosis. However, some people may have events that were not witnessed or that are more subtle, and establishing the diagnosis may require more steps. In this chapter, we will look at the process of how epilepsy is diagnosed and explore some other conditions that sometimes mimic epilepsy.

A clear understanding of the exact events that occur during a suspected seizure are very important for diagnosis, but your doctor will likely never see one of your seizures. For this reason, it is important for you and any observers of your events to provide as much detail as possible about what happened. The sequence of events—the "story"—is the basis of epilepsy diagnosis. Medical tests can help, but they do not replace a good seizure description. A clear diagnosis leads to good choices for treatment and will help your doctor tell you what to expect in the future.

Let's recall the definition of epilepsy from Chapter 2. In most cases a diagnosis of epilepsy is made when someone has had more than one unprovoked seizure, but remember—it is possible to establish a diagnosis of epilepsy after *only one* unprovoked seizure if the likelihood of having recurrent seizures is very high.

Before taking the next step down the path to epilepsy syndromes, it is important to first be clear that the episodes being addressed are in fact seizures. Often this may not be obvious. There is no simple blood test that can be used to determine whether someone has epilepsy. Seizures are brief, self-limited events and are unlikely to occur in the doctor's office. Therefore the diagnosis often rests heavily on a description of the event by friends, family, or bystanders, and, to a limited extent, from the patient himself.

Lee didn't think he had seizures or epilepsy. Lee was 52 and had been married to his wife Barbara for 22 years. She had recently observed some changes. The first time was 6 months ago when they were on vacation in Hawaii. They were getting ready to go to the beach, and she asked Lee if he had the keys to their condo. He didn't reply right away, and she found him sitting on the couch, looking at the bookcase. He had a "faraway look" in his eyes, and it took about 30 seconds for him to begin responding. He was then very concerned about where the dog was, apparently unaware that the dog was in the kennel back home in Illinois. Barbara had him lie down, and he fell asleep. After sleeping a couple of hours, he woke up and seemed to be himself again. They enjoyed a day at the beach and did not pursue a medical evaluation until this happened twice more: a second time at home after mowing the lawn, and then a third time while meeting with a colleague at work. His boss told him to go home for the rest of the day, and his co-worker suggested to his wife that they seek medical help. Their primary care provider was uncertain what was going on but arranged for Lee to see a neurologist. Lee thought that he was just "daydreaming," that he had a lot on his mind and that there was no need to "get all worked up over this." However, Barbara insisted that he see the neurologist.

Lee had two main questions:

1. What is going on/is there really anything wrong with me?
2. How will this affect my job?

Barbara added a third question to the list: Should Lee be driving?

Differential Diagnosis of Epilepsy

People don't come to their health care provider with a diagnosis of epilepsy. Instead, they are often having "episodes" or "spells"—periods of time where behavior or function is impaired, with relatively normal function before and after the episode. That was certainly the case with Lee.

When a patient comes in with "episodes," epilepsy is often a consideration, but it is usually one of several diagnoses being considered. In medical terminology, the doctor considers a variety of different reasons for the "episodes," called **differential diagnosis** (Box 6–1).

Syncope

Box 6–1 lists the main conditions that might imitate seizures. First on this list is **syncope**, which is the medical term for a fainting episode. Syncope occurs when the overall supply of blood and oxygen to the brain is temporarily interrupted. This could result from a sudden drop in blood pressure from a disturbance of the rhythm and pumping function of the heart or from a number of other causes. Syncope is a very common condition. You probably know someone who has fainted, or maybe you have experienced this yourself. The symptoms are often very characteristic. The earliest symptoms include feeling "faint" or lightheaded. You might feel a need to sit down or lower

---

BOX 6-1 Differential Diagnosis of Epilepsy in Adults

Syncope (fainting spells)
Transient ischemic attacks (TIAs, or "mini-strokes")
Sleep disorders
Migraine
Psychogenic nonepileptic seizures (PNES)

your head. Often this is accompanied by a feeling of nausea, darkening of the vision or seeing "spots," and a ringing in the ears. You might feel hot or sweaty. After a short time you might "pass out" or lose consciousness. This is usually brief and consists of a limp slumping to the ground. This is followed by restoration of blood flow to the brain and recovery. People who have experienced syncope are often uncertain about what just occurred, but they are generally not confused about their location or who familiar people around them are when they awaken. They may feel tired and "washed out," but they are usually able to function relatively well. In contrast, many seizures are followed by a period of greater confusion before recovery. This is a good example of why providing as much information to your doctor as possible about your events is important. A description of the typical presyncope feelings, the brief loss of consciousness with limp muscles, and the relatively rapid return to normal all help your doctor to suspect syncope instead of seizures.

A simple syncopal episode is not usually confused with a seizure. Uncertainty more often comes when the person experiencing syncope remains propped up in an upright position. Gravity can delay recovery of normal blood flow to the brain and lead to prolonged loss of consciousness. In this setting, it is not uncommon to have some stiffening or a few rhythmic jerks of the trunk or limbs. This is called **convulsive syncope** and can easily be mistaken for a seizure by untrained bystanders. Several times per year someone comes to our epilepsy clinic with a diagnosis of seizures, but with careful questioning an alternative diagnosis of convulsive syncope is made.

Transient Ischemic Attacks

Especially in older adults, a **transient ischemic attack (TIA)** may be mistaken for a seizure. A TIA is often thought of as a "mini-stroke." The symptoms are caused by blockage of blood flow to a specific part of the brain (as opposed to the global decrease in blood flow that occurs in syncope). This focal blockage of blood flow causes that area of the brain to not function normally. Usually this results in "negative symptoms"—a *loss* of function normally served by that brain area. This is in contrast to seizures, which often cause "positive symptoms"—those that result from *overactivity* in the brain region where the seizure occurs. A TIA in the motor control areas of the brain might cause weakness or paralysis on one side of the body, whereas a seizure in that same part of the brain might more likely cause stiffening or jerking of those body parts. TIAs generally last longer than seizures. However, there are exceptions to all of these rules. Since TIA is an episode that causes focal neurologic symptoms, it is easy to see how a TIA and seizure might be confused.

Sleep Disorders

Seizures can show many different patterns, and for some people, seizures may occur only at night, during sleep. Episodes that occur during the night can be difficult to diagnose. You might have no recall of them, and your bed partner may be asleep in the dark room and unable to describe them well. Not every nighttime episode is a seizure. Other sleep-related conditions include sleepwalking and related conditions, and **REM behavior disorder**, where people act out their dreams. Sometimes a detailed description and timing of the nighttime behavior leads to a clear diagnosis, but often additional testing is needed to distinguish nighttime seizures and sleep disorders.

Migraine

Next on the list is migraine. When people think of migraine, they usually think of a severe headache, which is often the main feature of migraine; however, other neurologic symptoms can occur, usually in the minutes just before headache onset. These symptoms are known as the migraine aura, which is different from a seizure aura. Visual auras are most common in migraine. These often include negative visual symptoms (a gradually enlarging blind spot) and positive visual symptoms (bright lights or jagged zigzag patterns, often at the edge of the blind spot). These visual symptoms gradually change or evolve over time and then often start to resolve as the headache begins. Some seizures that start in the visual areas of the brain can produce similar symptoms and make diagnosis difficult. Rarely, migraine auras can include temporary tingling, numbness, weakness, difficulty speaking, or other neurologic problems. Sometimes a headache does not follow these symptoms, and a seizure might be suspected.

A few other rare medical conditions can be imitators of seizures and epilepsy. These include myoclonic jerks that are not epileptic (see Chapter 2), and other brief movement disorders that are not connected to abnormal electrical discharges in the brain. In young children, the list is even longer and includes things like tics and breath-holding spells. Since this book focuses on adolescents and adults, we won't pursue this in more detail.

Taken together, the preceding list probably explains only one-tenth of the conditions that are mistaken for epilepsy. What makes up the other nine-tenths?

Psychogenic Nonepileptic Seizures

Psychogenic nonepileptic seizures (PNES) are seizure-like episodes that are *not* associated with an abnormal electrical discharge in the brain. In other words, the behavior observed can look similar to the behavior seen in someone having an epileptic seizure, but the cause is different. In PNES, the behavior is a physical change brought about by psychological or emotional stresses. How can underlying psychological stresses come out as seizure-like episodes?

If you think about it, you could probably list several physical symptoms that can be directly tied to emotional or psychological stresses—for example, headaches or an upset stomach. When we are embarrassed, we may blush—a physical change tied directly to emotions. PNES is another illustration of the strong mind–body connection.

Our understanding of PNES is still incomplete, and this category contains several different underlying conditions. The most common cause of PNES is felt to be **conversion disorder**. In conversion disorder, the theory is that a psychological trauma may reemerge, often years later, as a physical symptom. For example, a history of physical or sexual abuse is very common in people with PNES. Later in life, some of these earlier psychological stresses may reemerge as physical symptoms that may imitate medical conditions, especially neurologic ones.

The physical symptoms of a conversion disorder can take many forms, such as blindness, paralysis, or in this case, seizure-like behavior. In conversion disorder, there is no adequate medical explanation for the symptoms. The basis of the symptoms is psychological—but they are *very real* to the person who experiences them. Older terms for this condition, such as **hysterical seizures** or **pseudoseizures,** should be abandoned. They suggest that the person is "crazy" or "faking it," and both of these suggestions are incorrect. An individual experiencing a PNES generally has no more control over it than does a person with epilepsy over his or her seizures.

Laura is 51 and began experiencing convulsions two years earlier. Without any warning, she would suddenly slump to the ground and start shaking. Although she could not speak, she often retained some awareness of what was happening around her. Sometimes her left side would shake more and other times the right side. Sometimes the shaking would begin in one arm and move to the opposite leg. The convulsions sometimes lasted 10 to 15 minutes, and afterwards she was tired and would often cry. She had a history of two previous brief concussions. Her initial testing was inconclusive, and her doctor started her on an antiepileptic drug (AED).

(Continued)

(*Continued*)

Her convulsions improved for a few weeks, but then returned. Despite trying five other AEDs, alone and in combination, over the next 2 years, her convulsions persisted and became more frequent.

Things were not going well for Laura. While it was possible that Laura had epilepsy that was not responding to medications, her doctor had concerns about the diagnosis. He noted some unusual features of her events and referred her to an epilepsy center, where more detailed testing was performed and the correct diagnosis (PNES) was made.

Sometimes the diagnosis of PNES can be made in the neurologist's office, if the features are typical. More often, specialized testing, called video-EEG monitoring, is required to be certain. Video-EEG monitoring is discussed in Chapter 7. It is the "gold standard" for making a diagnosis of PNES. In a specialized hospital monitoring room, a video image and brain wave activity are recorded during a typical event, allowing a definite diagnosis.

At the epilepsy center, the diagnosis of PNES was explained to Laura carefully and thoughtfully. This allowed her to understand the diagnosis, and it did not make her feel bad or ashamed. She discovered that PNES is very common. Nearly one-third of patients who undergo video-EEG monitoring at some epilepsy centers actually have PNES and not epilepsy. It is more common in women than in men but is seen in both sexes. She learned that understanding and accepting the diagnosis is the first step toward controlling and eliminating PNES. She is now off of AEDs, which weren't helping her. She is receiving counseling from a mental health professional who is also treating her depression, which was identified in the course of her evaluation.

So PNES is a very important consideration in someone with seizure-like episodes. For those who would like to read more about PNES, please see Appendix 1 at the end of this book.

Chapter 7

Testing for Epilepsy

A detailed description of the seizure episodes is central to the process of making a diagnosis of epilepsy. We introduced Chapter 6 with the story of Lee and his wife Barbara. When Lee did see a neurologist, the detailed history that he and his wife were able to provide was extremely helpful for his neurologist, who was nearly certain that his spells represented seizures. He did order some additional tests to confirm the diagnosis.

Even though the history—the "story" of how the events unfold—is often most important, additional diagnostic testing is routinely performed and can play an important role. This testing might support the provisional diagnosis suggested by the description of the events. It might also suggest an alternative diagnosis. Additional testing can also help determine the epilepsy syndrome, which is very important for determining prognosis and treatment. It might also reveal the underlying *cause* of the epilepsy. In this chapter, we will learn more about the different medical tests that can help establish and refine the diagnosis of epilepsy. Some of these are very common tests that nearly everyone being evaluated for epilepsy will undergo. Others are used in more specialized circumstances.

Diagnostic testing for seizures and epilepsy falls into several categories, as noted in Box 7–1.

BOX 7-1 Diagnostic Tests for Seizures and Epilepsy

Laboratory testing
Electroencephalogram (EEG)
Brain imaging studies
    Magnetic resonance imaging (MRI)
    Computed tomography (CT)
Specialized testing

Laboratory Testing

If you have possible or known epilepsy, you have almost certainly had some laboratory or blood tests done. These tests are used in two ways. First, if you have known epilepsy and you are taking antiepileptic drugs (AEDs), blood tests are used to check the level of the medication in your bloodstream. This will be discussed in Chapter 10.

The second use of laboratory testing is to help with diagnosis—to identify abnormalities that might have produced the seizure. Most of this testing is done when epilepsy is first being investigated—for example, after you have had a first seizure.

Box 7–2 lists laboratory tests that are often considered after new-onset seizures. Not every test in Box 7–2 needs to be performed in every person. Doctors use their experience to select among these tests to best figure out what is wrong. Blood chemistry studies are used to look for imbalances in blood electrolytes (chemicals in the blood) that might cause seizures. These include both abnormally high or low levels of sodium, high or low levels of calcium, and high or low glucose (blood sugar). The complete blood count is used mostly to look for an elevation in the white blood cell count. White blood cells fight infection. If the level is high, it might trigger further search for infection. If there is concern about infection of the brain or the linings of the brain or spinal cord (encephalitis or meningitis), a lumbar

---

BOX 7-2 Laboratory Testing That Should Be Considered
in New-Onset Seizures

Blood chemistry studies
Complete blood count
Evaluation of spinal fluid
Urine screen for drugs of abuse
Prolactin level

---

puncture, or "spinal tap," might be performed. This is *not* done routinely in everyone with suspected seizures or epilepsy. It is reserved for times when there is high concern for brain infection.

In someone with new-onset seizures, the possibility of a provoked seizure from substance use is considered. Of greatest concern is abuse of stimulant medications such as methamphetamine or cocaine and withdrawal from alcohol or benzodiazepine medications such as diazepam (Valium) or its relatives. Other commonly used benzodiazepines include clonazepam (Klonopin) and lorazepam (Ativan). It is dangerous for someone who has been taking these medications regularly to stop them abruptly. Abrupt withdrawal can produce a number of symptoms, including seizures. Stopping alcohol after regular, heavy use can cause similar, very dangerous symptoms, including seizures.

A test to measure changes in the levels of a hormone called prolactin is not used very often, but if prolactin levels are checked immediately after a seizure, these findings might help your doctor decide whether or not you had a seizure.

Electroencephalography

Individuals being evaluated for seizures or epilepsy will likely undergo an electroencephalography (EEG) test. This is a fairly simple and painless test. The goal of the EEG test is to measure brain wave activity. An example of a normal EEG is shown in Figure 7–1. This picture is included just to give you an idea of what an EEG looks like. It takes years of training to learn how to interpret EEGs. A person with specialized training in performing EEG studies, called an EEG technologist, will gently cleanse the scalp and attach recording leads (small wires) at different points across the head. The leads are attached with a special paste. The hair is not cut or shaved, and the paste can be washed out after the test is completed. In some cases, the EEG study may be done as a sleep-deprived EEG. If this is the case, instructions will be given to stay up late the night before the EEG test and get very little sleep. This can help bring out abnormalities on the EEG and make it a more useful test.

During a routine EEG, individuals are asked to lie in a quiet room for 20 to 30 minutes while the recording is being obtained. The EEG machine simply records the electrical activity that is naturally occurring in the brain—there is no electricity applied to the head. The EEG technologist may ask you to breathe deeply and rapidly for a few minutes during the recording. They may also use a strobe light to expose you to flashing lights. Both of these measures make the EEG test more likely to detect helpful findings.

You may wonder what can be learned from a 30-minute EEG. There is almost no chance of recording a seizure in this short period of time. Instead, the goal is to make an **interictal** (between seizures) EEG recording. An interictal EEG can give doctors important clues that can support or clarify the diagnosis. Rarely, much longer EEG recordings are performed to obtain **ictal** (seizure) EEG recordings.

On an interictal EEG, there are several possible outcomes. First, the study could be completely normal. This does *not* mean that you have not experienced seizures or that you do not have epilepsy. Individuals with known epilepsy may have a completely normal routine EEG. Sometimes it is necessary to repeat a routine EEG, even several times, or to perform an extended EEG recording (see hereafter) to identify helpful abnormalities.

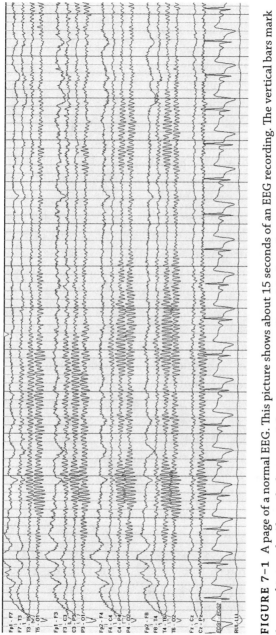

FIGURE 7–1 A page of a normal EEG. This picture shows about 15 seconds of an EEG recording. The vertical bars mark 1-second intervals. Along the bottom of the picture, a recording of the heartbeat is seen. All of the other lines represent the recording of brain wave activity from different locations on the scalp.

A second possible outcome of a routine EEG is that a nonspecific abnormality is found. It is not unusual that these relatively nonspecific abnormalities are seen, and your doctor will need to help you understand what they mean for you.

A third possible outcome on a routine EEG is detection of an abnormality that is much more specific for seizures and epilepsy. Since the routine EEG usually captures an interictal (between seizures) sample, the finding is not usually a seizure, but an interictal **epileptiform discharge**. These are usually called **spikes** or **sharp waves** (see Figure 7–2). They are not seizures, and they generally don't produce any symptoms that can be felt. They last for just a fraction of a second. They are electrical markers for seizures and epilepsy. Spikes and sharp waves are seen infrequently in people who don't have seizures. Rarely, someone who has a family member with epilepsy might show spikes or sharp waves on their EEG but might never experience seizures themselves. Thus a finding of an epileptiform discharge (spikes or sharp waves) is not 100 percent diagnostic of seizures, but it is strongly associated with seizures. In the right setting it can help increase our certainty about the diagnosis.

The finding of a specific epileptiform discharge on EEG goes beyond simply confirming the diagnosis. It can also help doctors diagnose the epilepsy syndrome (see Chapter 2). A doctor might find focal spikes on a person's EEG and decide that focal-onset seizures are occurring. The EEG might also provide some information about where in the brain the seizures start. Spikes that occur in both halves of the brain simultaneously suggest that the individual has a generalized epilepsy.

Figure 7–2 shows a focal epileptiform discharge. This finding is seen in someone who has focal-onset seizures. These include simple partial, complex partial, and secondarily generalized tonic-clonic seizures. You can refer to Chapter 2 or the Glossary if you'd like a reminder about the meaning of these seizure types. It is the most common epileptiform finding in adults with epilepsy.

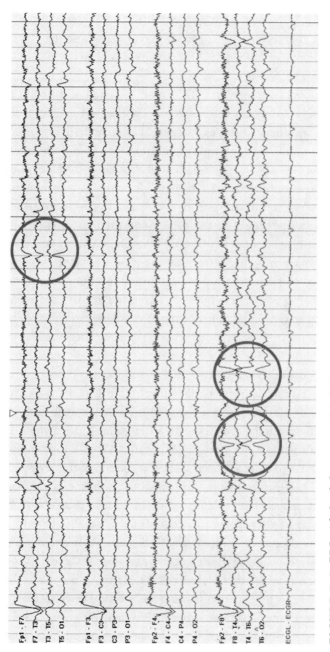

FIGURE 7-2 EEG with focal sharp waves (circled).

Figure 7–3 shows a run of generalized spike-wave activity. This suggests the presence of a generalized epilepsy and may be connected to one or several of the generalized seizure types discussed in Chapter 2.

In some cases, routine EEG, or even repeated routine EEGs, is not enough to obtain the necessary information needed to best manage epilepsy. At times, longer EEG recordings are needed. Sometimes this is simply an appointment for a longer EEG recording in the EEG lab—a 1- or 2-hour study instead of the more routine 20- to 30-minute recording. Increasingly common are **ambulatory EEG** studies. For an ambulatory EEG study, the leads are attached to the same positions on the head, but with a stronger glue that can hold the electrodes in place for 24 hours or more. The leads are attached to a pack that is worn on the waist. It is then possible to go home, do normal household activities, and then return to the EEG lab after 24 or more hours to have the EEG data downloaded and interpreted. In certain settings it can be very helpful to have information from an ambulatory EEG, which is recorded over an extended period, including during both wakefulness and sleep and during more normal activities. It allows more possibility of recording seizures and can be especially helpful for identifying or counting brief or subtle seizures or nighttime events. A small number of people may undergo even more extensive testing called **video-EEG monitoring** that takes place in the hospital. Video-EEG monitoring is discussed under specialized studies at the end of this chapter.

Thus EEG can be helpful for supporting a diagnosis of epilepsy and to establish the epilepsy syndrome. Most people with suspected seizures or epilepsy will undergo a routine EEG, but at times it may be necessary to repeat the EEG study or do extended EEG recordings to establish the diagnosis or syndrome. Once these goals have been reached, there is generally little to no benefit in doing repeated EEGs to "see what is going on." Because each EEG looks at just a short sample of time, a routine EEG may vary from normal to abnormal on different days. Therefore in someone with established

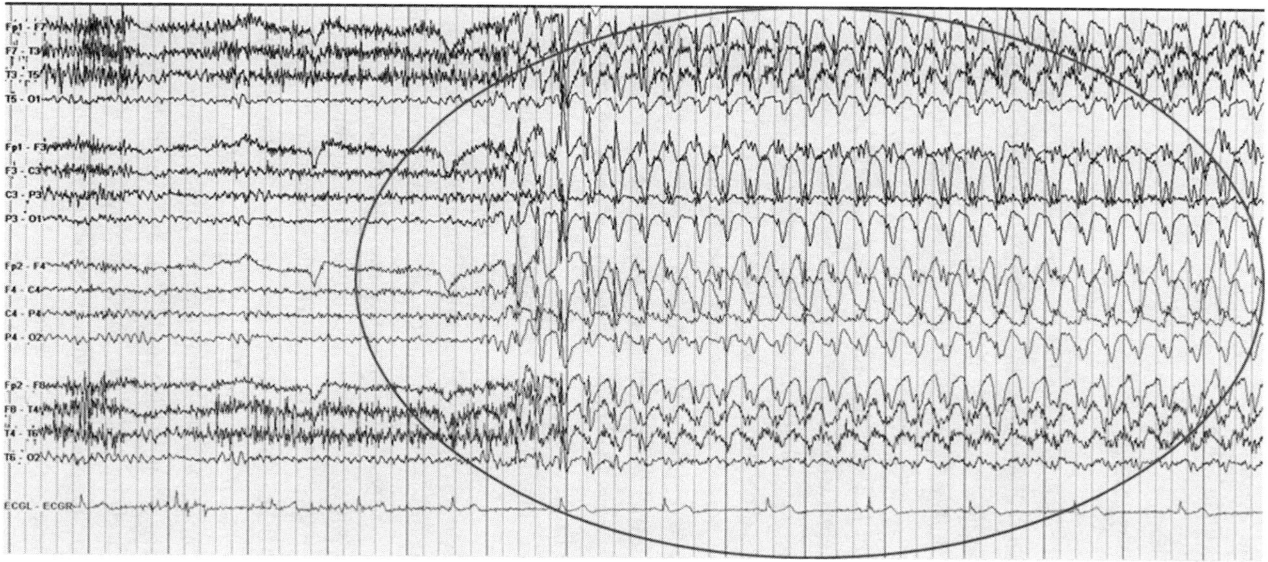

FIGURE 7-3 EEG with generalized spike wave discharges (within large circle).

epilepsy and an identified epilepsy syndrome diagnosis, repeated EEGs are of little value.

Brain Imaging

When someone is suspected of having a seizure or epilepsy, a brain imaging test will probably be ordered if it has not been done previously. The goal is to see if an abnormality in the brain can be identified that is responsible for the seizures. In the emergency department setting, after a first seizure, it is likely that a **computed tomography (CT or CAT)** scan of the head will be done. CT scanning is widely available, fast, and can be performed even in people who may be somewhat confused and not following directions well. It gives a reasonably good picture of the brain and can evaluate for some of the causes of seizures that need immediate attention, such as bleeding in or around the brain and large masses or tumors.

If a CT scan did not identify any important findings in the urgent setting, it is most likely that a **magnetic resonance imaging (MRI)** scan of the brain will be requested.

Why should an MRI scan be performed in someone who has a normal head CT scan? The reason is that the MRI produces much more detailed pictures of the brain. Numerous studies have shown that MRI is much better than CT at detecting brain abnormalities that cause seizures. Sometimes the findings are subtle—a small area of scarring in the brain from a prior head injury, or a tiny focal area where the brain didn't form normally during brain development. However, MRI can also detect abnormalities missed by CT that not only cause seizures, but might also require additional attention. For example, some low-grade, slow-growing tumors are not well seen on CT scan but are easily seen on MRI. If discovered, these need to be watched closely by repeated scans or sometimes surgically removed. Some malformations of blood vessels in the brain can cause seizures. Many of these are much better seen on MRI than CT scan. Some of these blood vessel malformations pose a high risk of bleeding and may require additional attention, including surgery in some cases. The added diagnostic ability of the MRI leads to better treatment of epilepsy and related conditions, in many cases.

Not all MRI scans are the same, however. Some recent studies have suggested that both the quality of the MRI scanner and the experience of the physician reading the scan play a big part in determining whether a cause of seizures is identified. If possible, MRI scans should be done at a center that is experienced in epilepsy care, especially if the seizures have been difficult to control. Ask your doctor if you need a referral to an experienced epilepsy center.

Martin was 37 years old. He had his first seizure at age 25, and he was diagnosed with epilepsy that same year. He had never experienced seizures as a child, and he did not seem to have any risk factors for developing epilepsy. His EEG showed spikes in the right frontal lobe, but his MRI scan was normal at the time of diagnosis. It was suspected that his seizures might be coming from the region of the right frontal lobe, but he was told that he fell into the fairly large group of patients in whom no cause for the epilepsy could be found.

His seizures were never well controlled by antiepileptic drugs. By age 35, 10 years had elapsed since his first MRI scan was done, and the technology had advanced tremendously. His neurologist sent him for a repeat MRI scan of the brain, which was performed at an epilepsy center with state-of-the art MRI scanners and experienced readers of the images (neuroradiologists). The repeat MRI scan was finally able to answer why Martin has epilepsy. A small malformation that occurs during brain development called a **focal cortical dysplasia** was found in Martin's right frontal lobe. Because of his poor seizure control over the preceding 10 years, Martin and his neurologist

(Continued)

(Continued)
pursued further testing for epilepsy surgery (see Chapter 11). The seizure focus, including the cortical dysplasia, was safely removed surgically, and Martin has been seizure free for the past 2 years. MRI certainly made a tremendous difference in Martin's life.

Specialized Testing

This section provides an introduction to some of the other specialized testing that can be used to evaluate people with epilepsy. Most people with epilepsy do not undergo all of these tests. In general, they are used to evaluate people with very difficult-to-control seizures who may be considering epilepsy surgery. In the case of video-EEG monitoring, the testing can also be used to clarify the diagnosis.

Video-EEG Monitoring

Video-EEG monitoring was mentioned earlier in the EEG section. This is a specialized form of EEG testing that is performed in a select group of people. The main reasons for doing this test are:

- To establish a diagnosis for someone with "episodes" or "spells" when standard testing is unable to do so
- To record seizures and locate the brain region where seizures begin as a step on the path to epilepsy surgery
- To clarify the epilepsy syndrome or quantify (count) subtle seizures

Let's examine these one at a time, beginning with use of video-EEG to clarify diagnosis.

Anna was 17 years old and by all measures very successful. She was a straight-A student, one of the stars of the soccer team, and very involved in theater. She was well liked and had a circle of friends she enjoyed spending time with. Her first episode occurred during a rehearsal for the school play. She was on stage, in the middle of her lines, when she suddenly collapsed, stiffened, and had whole-body shaking. These episodes became repetitive, occurring about once per week, and quickly grew to dominate her life. Her parents, understandably concerned, took Anna to her primary care provider and then quickly to a neurologist. The neurologist suspected seizures based on the description, although the MRI and routine EEG were normal. The events persisted despite trials of two different antiepileptic drugs, and she was referred for video-EEG monitoring to establish a definitive diagnosis.

Most epilepsy diagnosis is done in the clinic. Through the process just described, a careful medical history and description of the events, a neurologic examination, and supportive testing is usually sufficient to arrive at a firm diagnosis of epilepsy or one of the alternative diagnoses. In some cases, however, the diagnosis may still be unclear. In this situation, some doctors may proceed with a *therapeutic trial*. In other words, they may prescribe an AED because they believe epilepsy is the best fit for the symptoms. If the episodes stop, this is taken as support that epilepsy was the correct diagnosis. Often this can be a difficult approach. If there appears to be an initial response and then a return of the episodes, what can be concluded? Is it epilepsy that showed an incomplete response to the first medication tried? Is the epilepsy diagnosis incorrect? Drawing conclusions from therapeutic trials can be difficult, and the diagnostic waters are often muddy. In Anna's case, there did not seem to be any response to the therapeutic trial. If the episodes are fairly frequent, video-EEG monitoring can help arrive at a definitive diagnosis.

As the name suggests, the test is a combination of video—a visual recording of what happens during an episode—and EEG—a brain wave recording *during* the episode of interest. This testing is performed in a specialized hospital room, usually at an epilepsy center, and usually over a period of several days. The EEG electrodes are attached to the scalp using a special type of glue, and EEG technologists check and repair the electrodes on at least a daily basis. A small video camera is mounted in the room so a video image of any episodes can be captured.

If the episodes are very frequent, the testing may consist mostly of observation and recording of the events. More commonly, measures are taken to encourage episodes to occur. AEDs may be reduced or discontinued. Other common measures include staying up late and getting little sleep (sleep deprivation). This can help bring out abnormalities on the EEG or trigger episodes. Other measures include rapid deep breathing (hyperventilation) and flashing strobe lights (photic stimulation). If a particular trigger for seizures has been identified, that might be employed, if practical. Often it is helpful, if possible, to record more than one of the typical events.

Anna had two of her typical events during 3 days of video-EEG monitoring. Her EEG was entirely normal throughout the 3 days. Her neurologist was able to view the video and the EEG recorded during the events. There were no EEG changes during the events, and the video showed features strongly associated with **psychogenic nonepileptic events (PNES)**. On further questioning, there was significant conflict in the home, as the parents were in the process of separating. Anna was taken off of AED therapy, was referred for psychological counseling, and did extremely well. Her episodes are now a thing of the past.

In most cases, a definitive diagnosis can be reached by the end of a video-EEG monitoring stay. This can often provide a useful "short-cut" to receiving the proper treatment. For those with a diagnosis of nonepileptic events, it can limit lengthy and potentially risky treatment trials with AEDs, which are ineffective in nonepileptic events. It can help redirect therapy to addressing the underlying (nonepileptic) problem. For those with epilepsy, it can confirm the diagnosis and syndrome and suggest useful paths of treatment. Overall, the information obtained is often very useful for making treatment decisions and helps avoid some of the "trial-and-error" approach.

Let's look at some other examples of how video-EEG monitoring can be useful.

Mark and Phillip happened to undergo video-EEG monitoring in the same week. They both had epilepsy that had not responded to several trials of AEDs, and the goal for both of them was the same: to explore whether they might be candidates for epilepsy surgery. Both underwent testing in a specialized video-EEG monitoring unit, both had their AEDs safely reduced, and several seizures were recorded for each of them. The outcomes, however, were quite different. Mark's video-EEG captured five seizures, all of which arose from the temporal lobe on the right. He had previously undergone a brain MRI that showed a likely seizure focus in the right temporal lobe. His epilepsy care team told him that a few more tests were needed, but that the video-EEG monitoring showed encouraging findings and a potentially curative epilepsy surgery procedure might likely be possible.

Phillip's video-EEG recorded six seizures during his stay. He was also found to have temporal lobe epilepsy, but unlike Mark, three of his seizures started in the left temporal region, while three others began in the right temporal region. Because

(Continued)

(*Continued*)

seizures started independently in both temporal lobes, his epilepsy care team told him it would not be safe to remove both areas. Phillip was disappointed, but felt satisfied that he had explored the possibility of surgery thoroughly and now knew that that option was off the table. He continued working with his team to explore other medication options and to discuss the possibility of using medical devices to treat his epilepsy (see Chapter 12).

Sometimes video-EEG monitoring is useful in different ways.

Ashley was 27 years old when she first had video-EEG monitoring. She had known epilepsy and had previously experienced complex partial and secondarily generalized seizures. She had tried two different AEDs, and the second seemed to work well. She had no definite daytime complex partial or secondarily generalized seizures. Yet she was still concerned that sometimes she would "space out" during the day, and at times she would also feel very tired on waking in the morning and wondered if she might be having undetected nighttime seizures. The purpose of Ashley's video-EEG monitoring was not to establish the diagnosis (she had known epilepsy) or for presurgical evaluation (she did not need epilepsy surgery), but rather to clarify whether she was having ongoing subtle seizures. Ashley and her family were relieved that no evidence of active seizures was found during her 4 days of video-EEG monitoring. The team did discover that she had trouble with breathing during sleep (sleep apnea), and effective treatment of her sleep disorder improved all of her symptoms.

So to summarize: Only a small subset of people with epilepsy need video-EEG monitoring. This form of testing is most useful to:

- Establish a diagnosis for someone with "episodes" or "spells" when usual means are unable to do so
- Record seizures and locate the brain region where seizures begin as a step on the path to epilepsy surgery
- Clarify the epilepsy syndrome or quantify (count) subtle seizures

Intracranial EEG

An even smaller number of patients may need intracranial EEG recordings. They are used only in people who are on a path to epilepsy surgery.

Sometimes standard EEG recordings with electrodes attached to the scalp do not provide enough detail to locate the seizure focus. The scalp is separated from the brain regions of interest by the skull, spinal fluid, and coverings of the brain. All of these barriers affect the EEG signal and can make it harder to locate a seizure focus.

With **intracranial EEG**, a neurosurgeon places the electrodes directly on the surface of the brain or within the brain. This is done in the operating room under general anesthesia (the patient is asleep).

There are several types of intracranial electrodes, and each serves a different purpose and requires a slightly different procedure. **Depth electrodes** (Figure 7–4) look like very thin spears. Along each spear are several electrode contacts. Often several depth electrodes are placed to sample the electrical activity from different areas of the brain. These are inserted by the neurosurgeon through small holes in the skull so that they are positioned in or near the seizure focus. With the use of an image-guided navigation system in the operating

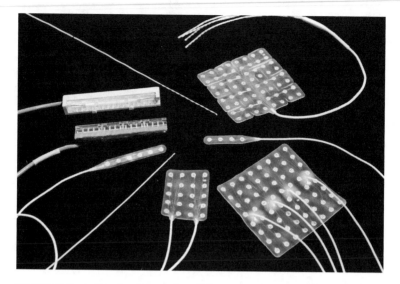

FIGURE 7-4 Depth, strip, and grid electrodes. Image courtesy Ad-Tech medical instrument corporation.

room, the placement of these electrodes can be quite precise. These are the only electrodes that can record from within the brain itself, and are useful for recording from deep structures. **Strip electrodes** consist of several thin, flat recording disks embedded in a flexible, clear plastic strip. Strip electrodes are also inserted through holes, but these are larger (the size of a quarter). Sometimes several strips can be inserted through each hole, with each strip oriented in a different direction. **Grid electrodes** are square or rectangular arrays of thin, flat recoding electrodes embedded in a flexible plastic sheet. Surgical placement of grid electrodes requires the most extensive procedure. Under general anesthesia, the surgeon removes a section of the skull, places the electrode grid on the surface of the brain, and replaces the skull. This can sound scary, but it is a procedure with which surgeons at an epilepsy center will be very experienced. The information obtained from the use of grid electrodes can sometimes be the critical piece that allows epilepsy surgery to go forward successfully. They are very useful when the general area of seizure onset is known but fine detail is needed. The closely spaced electrodes allow for careful mapping of the seizure-onset zone, providing the epilepsy surgeon with critical information about the exact area of seizure onset.

The exact pattern or array of intracranial electrodes is tailored for each person. After electrode placement, patients are brought to an epilepsy monitoring unit with video-EEG monitoring that is specialized for intracranial electrode recording. Following these recordings, the patient returns to the operating room for removal of the intracranial electrodes, and surgery to resect, or cut out, the seizure focus, if indicated.

Intracranial electrodes—especially grids—can have a second purpose: **brain mapping** (also known as **cortical stimulation mapping**). This can be important when the seizure focus is near an area of critical brain function. Brain mapping can determine the function of the brain tissue that lies under the grid. The brain tissue that lies under the grid is stimulated by passing a weak electrical current through one of the grid electrodes (controlled by the neurologist). This briefly affects the function of that small area of the brain. For example, if this is an area related to sight, some spots might appear in the patient's vision. If the area is concerned with movement, a finger or arm might move. The areas of the brain being stimulated do not have sensory nerve endings (they can't "feel"), so the stimulation is not felt in the head. By passing a weak current through each electrode on the grid, the neurologist can create a map of the function of the brain underneath the grid. The epilepsy surgeon can use this map to avoid removing any brain tissue that serves a critical function.

Intracranial electrode testing carries possible risks, including bleeding, stroke, or infection. Overall the risks are relatively small, but they can be very serious if they do occur. It is important to have a discussion with your doctor of the risks and benefits of intracranial EEG monitoring in advance of the procedure.

Positron Emission Tomography

Positron emission tomography (PET) is a special type of picture of the brain. This test is not done routinely in people with epilepsy. It is usually reserved for a select group of patients who are undergoing evaluation for epilepsy surgery.

Whereas MRI produces an image of the *structure* of the brain, a PET scan provides a picture of the *function* of the brain. When used in epilepsy, PET images usually give us a picture of how much sugar each part of the brain is using as fuel. Put another way, the PET scan looks at brain metabolism. All brain cells use sugar as fuel, but areas of the brain that are not working properly will use less sugar than healthy areas. Even if a part of the brain looks normal on MRI, it may still not be functioning correctly, and this can be seen on the PET scan. Areas of the brain that are not functioning correctly (called "hypometabolic") often turn out to be the parts of the brain that generate seizures.

PET scans are especially helpful when the location of the seizure focus is uncertain, even after video-EEG monitoring and MRI. Identification of a hypometabolic area can sometimes be a critical piece of epilepsy surgery planning.

PET scans are performed in a nuclear medicine laboratory. The patient is given an intravenous (IV) injection of a "tracer," in this case a radioactive sugar (also called a radionuclide). The dose of radiation is extremely small and of no harm to the body. This tracer circulates through the blood and into the brain, and is taken up by brain cells to use as fuel. The patient then lies on a table while a scanner counts the small amount of radioactivity coming from different parts of the brain and assembles this into a picture. Usually the scanning procedure lasts from 30 to 60 minutes.

Single-Photon Emission Computed Tomography

Single-photon emission computed tomography (SPECT), like PET, is a nuclear medicine study that is a specialized test sometimes used in patients undergoing evaluation for epilepsy surgery. It is not a routine test for most people with epilepsy.

In contrast to PET, which uses a tracer that measures the use of sugar in the brain, SPECT scans use a tracer that tracks *blood flow* to different parts of the brain. As with PET, a patient may come in to the nuclear medicine laboratory for this test, where an IV injection of a "tracer" is given. In this case, the radioactive tag is taken up by brain cells based on how much blood flow they receive. The dose of radiation is extremely small and of no harm to the body. The patient then lies on a table while a scanner counts the small amount of radioactivity coming from different parts of the brain and assembles this into a picture. When a seizure is not occurring, the area of a seizure focus may receive less blood flow than other parts of the brain. Used in this way, SPECT may identify a seizure focus not seen on MRI, but it is less sensitive than PET. However, there is a second use for SPECT that can be much more powerful.

Because the tracer for SPECT remains active for several hours, it can be kept near the patient and then injected *during* a seizure (an "ictal SPECT"). During a seizure, there is increased activity of the brain cells at the seizure focus. This results in increased blood flow to that area, which can be measured with a SPECT scan. Getting the timing right to successfully inject the tracer during a seizure is challenging, but a successful SPECT test can be extremely helpful in locating the seizure-onset zone.

For someone who is having very frequent seizures, it is possible that an ictal SPECT could be done in the nuclear medicine laboratory. More often it is done during video-EEG monitoring. With both video and EEG being recorded, the epilepsy team watches the patient carefully, and when a seizure occurs the team rapidly responds by giving the SPECT tracer. The blood flow changes with a seizure are temporary, so the goal is to perform the injection as soon as possible, ideally within 30 seconds of the seizure onset. With this injection, a "snapshot" of the blood flow to the brain at that point in time is taken, and the tracer remains stable in the brain for a period of a couple of hours. This allows a reasonable timeframe for the actual SPECT scan to be performed after the injection is complete.

One more processing step is often performed that makes the ictal SPECT scan especially useful. This is sometimes called **SISCOM (subtraction ictal SPECT coregistered to MRI)**. That is a mouthful, so you can see why it is called SISCOM for short! In this process, the patient has two SPECT scans, one *during* a seizure (ictal SPECT) and one *in between* seizures (interictal SPECT). The two images are lined up and subtracted from each other. What remains is the difference between the ictal and interictal SPECT scans. Remember, the interictal SPECT may show low blood flow at the seizure focus, and the ictal SPECT shows high blood flow at the focus. Brain regions outside of the seizure focus usually don't show changes in blood flow. Thus the subtraction will ideally "light up" the area of blood flow changes between the interictal and ictal studies—the seizure focus. The result is then overlaid on the patient's MRI scan so the location of the focus can be easily seen.

Undergoing SPECT and SISCOM can be an involved process that is difficult to successfully complete, but these tests can be powerful tools to identify a seizure focus, especially when the MRI shows no seizure focus or more than one possible area for it.

Magnetoencephalography

Magnetoencephalography (MEG) is related to EEG but is not a routine test for most people with epilepsy. Instead, it is another of the tests that is usually reserved for people undergoing an epilepsy surgery evaluation.

EEG detects the electrical activity of the brain through electrodes temporarily attached to the scalp. MEG does not directly measure the electrical activity of the brain, but instead measures the small magnetic fields created by the brain's electrical activity. Like EEG, it can detect spikes and sharp waves that often occur in or near a seizure focus.

MEG has several advantages over EEG and other ways of identifying a seizure focus (PET, SPECT). It is noninvasive and painless, and no radioactive materials have to be given. The MEG signals are not distorted by the coverings of the brain and the skull as with EEG. The greater detail obtained can be an advantage when trying to pinpoint the source of epileptic activity. It looks at the seizure focus in a different way from these other tests and thus may provide complementary information. The main disadvantage of MEG is that the equipment is much larger and more expensive than that used for EEG, and the recording time is limited. MEG is also more limited in its ability to locate a seizure focus deep in the brain.

The MEG recording machine looks very different from an EEG machine. The patient is seated in a chair or may be lying on a semi-reclined couch. All metal must be removed from the patient to avoid interference with the sensitive detectors in the machine. The MEG machine is a large unit, with a helmet-shaped space for the patient's head. This helmet contains the magnetic detectors capable of mea-suring tiny magnetic fields. The remainder of the procedure is much like any EEG recording. The patient simply sits quietly for about 30 to 60 minutes while brain waves are recorded. Brain waves are then computer-analyzed to produce a map of magnetic-electrical activity in the brain. This map can be displayed directly on the MRI to show the source of electrical activity related to seizures.

MEG is often used in situations where EEG activity is difficult to localize and where this information is critical to the presurgical evaluation. As with all epilepsy surgery tests, the epilepsy care team must consider the results of MEG in combination with the results of other studies. Agreement between several tests greatly improves the chances of a successful surgical outcome (Chapter 11).

Functional Magnetic Resonance Imaging

Functional MRI (fMRI) is a special type of MRI scan that can help identify brain regions that serve important functions. This is not a routine test for people with epilepsy but is usually reserved for those undergoing epilepsy surgery. The goal of fMRI is usually to identify these critical brain regions so they can be spared during a surgery to remove the seizure focus.

A standard MRI machine can be used to perform fMRI, but the way the images are obtained is different. The person undergoing fMRI is asked to perform a specific task. If motor areas of the brain are being mapped, they may be asked to do repeated finger tapping. For language areas, tasks such as thinking of a word might be used. Computer processing of the images obtained creates a map of areas active for that function to be overlaid on top of the picture of the brain. The surgeon can then use this information for presurgical planning. Another, slightly related MRI technique called **diffusion tensor imaging (DTI)** may also be used in a similar manner to map the pathways in the white matter (wiring of the brain) to be avoided during surgery.

Wada Test, or Intracarotid Amobarbital Procedure

The **Wada test,** or **intracarotid amobarbital procedure** (IAP), are two names for the same test. Here it will be referred to as the Wada test, as that term is most commonly used. This test is done only in select patients prior to epilepsy surgery.

First, an **angiogram** is performed. An angiogram is a test in which a dye is put into an artery and X-ray pictures of the blood vessels of the brain are taken. Next, a short-acting medication called amobarbital is given to one-half of the brain that essentially "puts half of the brain to sleep" for about 10 minutes. During that time, tests of language and memory are given. After recovery, the other half of the brain is put to sleep, and testing is repeated. At the end of the test, the examiner can tell which half of the brain is most important for language function. Important information about memory function is also gained. The epilepsy surgery team can then use this information to help make sure a planned surgery is as safe as possible by avoiding risks to language and memory function. As fMRI has become better developed, it can be used in place of the Wada test in some cases.

Neuropsychological Testing

A final specialized test that is usually part of a presurgical evaluation (and that is not performed in most people with epilepsy) is neuro-psychological testing. This testing consists of a battery of tests of cognitive (thinking) and psychological/emotional function. These are "pencil and paper" tests that assess memory, language, spatial skills, problem solving, processing speed, and other cognitive skills. Some of the interview and testing also addresses emotional and psychological functioning.

This information can be used in the presurgical assessment in several ways. First, it establishes a baseline for thinking abilities that can serve as a comparison if there are any concerns following surgery. Second, the pattern of strengths and weaknesses may help identify parts of the brain that are involved with seizures. This pattern might also point out if there are any particular risks to cognitive function from the planned surgery. Finally, it might help identify depression or other psychological issues that need to be addressed before consideration of epilepsy surgery.

Neuropsychological testing also has a role outside of epilepsy surgery, and the information gained from this testing can help address concerns about memory and other cognitive or psycho-logical functioning in people who are not undergoing epilepsy surgery.

Genetic Testing

Most of the specialized or nonroutine tests that we have discussed are different ways to image or measure brain activity. However, another important emerging area is genetic testing.

In Chapter 5 we discussed genetic forms of epilepsy. We learned that a tiny fraction of genetic epilepsy is caused by a simple defect in a single gene. For the vast majority of genetic epilepsies, the problem is polygenic—small changes in multiple genes add up to produce or contribute to epilepsy.

Our scientific understanding of the complex genetics of epilepsy has grown rapidly in the last 5 to 10 years. However, a large gap remains between the science and what can be practically tested for in the clinic. This gap is likely to close rapidly in the next several years as the technology improves and as we are better able to interpret the huge streams of data that come from testing a person's entire genome.

At the present time, most genetic testing falls into the category of "specialized" testing that is not used routinely in most patients with seizures or epilepsy. For now, it is important to be aware of two areas of genetic testing

Genetic Testing for Diagnosis of Epilepsy Syndrome

Presently, genetic testing for diagnosis of an epilepsy syndrome is very limited. The people who are most likely to benefit from a search for a known single gene defect are infants and young children with severe forms of epilepsy. Genetic testing in the clinic has begun to come into more widespread use for this group, and there are indications that it can identify the cause of epilepsy in a substantial number of children in whom the cause had not previously been identified. For most everyone else, and for most adults with epilepsy, genetic testing is low yield and not likely to produce findings that help with diagnosis or treatment. This is clearly an area where research and technology have outpaced our understanding of human epilepsy. It is becoming increasingly feasible to learn one's entire genetic sequence—even with a mail order test—but at the present time we don't know how to interpret many of the findings, and such testing often raises more questions than it answers.

Pharmacogenomics

Pharmacogenomics is another branch of genetics that is concerned with how our genes determine our responses to medications. Why do some people develop a rash as an allergic response to a particular medication? Why does a medication work well for one patient but not seem to help another at all? Some, or at times much, of this variation is due to genetics. The pharmacogenomics of epilepsy is being actively investigated but is still in its infancy.

At the present time, there is limited use of genetic testing to determine risk of allergic reaction to certain seizure medications.

Perhaps one day a person with new-onset epilepsy will take a blood test that determines that she will have a bad reaction to two AEDs, and that seizures will likely not respond to three others, thus narrowing the medication selection and bypassing a great deal of trial and error.

We are not there yet, but in future editions of the book, I expect genetic testing may move from the current position as "specialized testing" to become a routine test like EEG or MRI that is performed in most people with suspected seizures or epilepsy.

Chapter 8

Treatment of Epilepsy

Overview of Epilepsy Treatment

Treatment of epilepsy is a big topic. In fact, it is such a big topic that it is the focus of the rest of the chapters in this book. Let's start with an overview of the topics that will be covered and the questions that will be answered in the next five chapters.

This chapter introduces some of the "big picture" ideas with regard to treatment, including the following:

- The decision to start treatment: Who needs to go on treatment to prevent further seizures? When is an approach of "watchful waiting" more appropriate?
- Nonpharmacological treatment: What nonmedication approaches can everyone benefit from to help prevent seizures?
- Stopping AEDs: When, if ever, is it safe to discontinue AED therapy?

If you look ahead to the upcoming chapters that also address treatment, you will encounter:

- Chapter 9: Antiepileptic Drug Therapy. Because so many different medications are available, this section could easily become far too long. The chapter includes a list of commonly used medications, but then focuses on several specific areas:

- Antiepileptic drug (AED) mechanisms: How do they work?
- Basic principles of AED selection: What is the best AED for you? How is this decided? When is single-drug therapy adequate, and when should AEDs be used in combination? I will specifically avoid going through each medication and listing lots of facts. That could quickly become overwhelming. However, in Appendix 2, you will find some additional detail on specific medications as a reference.

- Chapter 10: Side Effects. This chapter covers common medication side effects and answers the following questions: What medication side effects should you watch for when starting on AED therapy? Why are these so important? A way to organize and review the common side effects of antiepileptic medications will be discussed. Appendix 2 lists some of the more common side effects seen with certain specific medications, and can be used as a reference if you want more information about a specific medication you are taking.

Chapter 10 will also review two important topics with regard to AED side effects:

- AED interactions: What AEDs should not be used together because of negative drug interactions? Which ones work well together? What interactions can there be between AEDs and other drugs? Again, this section will focus on general principles and will try to avoid being a "laundry list" of every potential drug–drug interaction known. Appendix 2 will highlight some important interactions of specific medications.
- AED monitoring: How and when should AED levels and other blood tests to monitor medications be performed?

- Moving beyond AED therapy, several important topics are covered in Chapters 11 and 12.
  - Chapter 11: Beyond AEDs: Surgical Therapies. When should epilepsy surgery be considered? What are the different types of epilepsy surgery? How safe and effective is epilepsy surgery?
  - Chapter 12: Beyond AEDs: Other Therapeutic Options. This chapter covers three important areas:
    - Medical devices: When should you consider use of a medical device to treat your epilepsy?
    - Complementary and alternative medications: You may have heard about other approaches outside of conventional medicine to treat epilepsy. Should these be considered? Should you tell your doctor if you are already using some? This chapter will cover what we know and what we still need to know.
    - Dietary therapy: Have you thought about using a special diet to treat your epilepsy? What diets are safe and effective in adolescents and adults?
- Chapter 13: Treatment in Special Populations and Situations. We wrap up the treatment theme in Chapter 13, where treatment in special populations is addressed:
  - What special treatment considerations do women need to be aware of?
  - Should treatment be different if you are older?
  - What is different for teens with epilepsy?
  - How should treatment be tailored if you have had unusually long seizures?

For now, let's start at the beginning, and look at when treatment is needed.

The Decision to Start Treatment

Matt was 30 years old when he experienced his first seizure. He had just returned to the United States from a business trip to Asia, which he did several times per year. Although he had not been feeling well, he hadn't wanted to disappoint his hosts, who took him out for a "going away" celebration the night before his departure. He had several alcoholic drinks that night and slept poorly before his early-morning flight home. When he arrived home, he was exhausted, and he fell asleep on his couch. His girlfriend, Crystal, was in the room with him and heard him cry out and then stiffen. He didn't seem to be breathing, and his lips looked a little blue. She didn't know what was happening and thought maybe he was having a stroke. She called 911, and while she talked to them, Matt started having rhythmic whole-body jerking that then stopped, leaving him unresponsive but breathing. The entire seizure lasted a little less than a minute, but it seemed like forever to Crystal. Matt woke to find that both his tongue, which he had bitten during the episode, and his whole body were very sore. He was confused, but he recalled the trip to the emergency department. His neurologic examination and laboratory testing were normal, and he later had an EEG and brain MRI that were also normal. Matt was otherwise healthy, and he found the whole experience unsettling and somewhat frightening. He definitely did *not* want to ever go through that again. Matt's neurologist confirmed that he had, indeed, experienced a generalized tonic-clonic seizure. Among the many questions he had for his neurologist was this: "Do I need to go on a seizure medication to prevent future seizures?"

Everyone who has experienced a seizure has his or her own unique circumstances. Although everyone is different, each person and his or her doctor will have to consider the same questions. A central question will be, "What is the risk of having another seizure?" If the risk of recurrence is felt to be high, the neurologist will probably recommend AED therapy.

Why shouldn't everyone who has had a seizure go on AED treatment? If AEDs were 100 percent effective, free of any side effects, and free of cost, that might be a consideration. While AEDs are very useful, safe, and effective in the right situation, they can certainly also have side effects, which are discussed in greater detail in Chapter 10. Therefore AEDs should be used selectively. If the risk of recurrent seizures is low, it is likely that your doctor may say that AEDs are not appropriate right now.

The decision of what steps to take after a *provoked* seizure is often more straightforward.

Bill was 72 years old when he was hospitalized with a serious illness that caused his kidneys to stop functioning and affected many other organ systems. He was in the intensive care unit (ICU) of the hospital for two weeks before his condition stabilized enough for him to be discharged to a rehabilitation facility. During the most severe phase of his illness he was quite sick. His kidneys weren't doing their usual job of clearing waste products from the bloodstream, his blood sodium and calcium levels were outside of the normal range, and he was told that he had had a seizure. He recalled nothing about it. His doctors thought the seizure was provoked by his severe kidney disease and disturbed blood sodium and calcium levels. These problems subsequently resolved. He was no longer at risk for a provoked seizure, and his doctor told him that he did not need to start AED therapy. His seizure risk was now not much different from that of the general population.

Decisions about AED therapy may also be relatively straightforward if a person has had *more than one unprovoked* seizure. By definition, more than one unprovoked seizure is epilepsy, and treatment with AEDs is usually what most doctors will recommend. But why is this the case? We need to go back to the question that guides the decision to initiate treatment: What is the risk of recurrence? After two unprovoked seizures, the risk that a third or fourth seizure will happen is quite high—around 70 to 80 percent in most studies. Given those odds and the risk of injury or harm that could come from further seizures, most doctors recommend (and most individuals want) treatment to reduce the risk of having more seizures.

There are some gray areas. What if the two unprovoked seizures happened 15 years apart? Does it make sense to take a daily AED to prevent something that might not happen again for another 15 to 20 years? What if the symptoms of the seizure were very mild—for example, two simple partial seizures with mild twitching of the fingers? In these gray areas, it is best to have a detailed discussion with your doctor about the risks and benefits of treatment or no treatment. The decision making needs to be individualized to the specific circumstances, and it is not possible to make a single recommendation for all.

Judging the Risk of Recurrence

Let's return to Matt's situation to consider decision making after a single seizure. Although some factors in Matt's history might have explained why the seizure occurred on the day that it did (alcohol use, sleep deprivation), none of these factors was strong enough to cause the seizure by itself. Many people are in similar circumstances every day and do not have seizures. Thus Matt's seizure cannot be considered a provoked seizure.

The need to make a decision about whether to start an AED after a single seizure is common. Doctors want to have good data on the risk of having more seizures to aid with decision making. Fortunately, several large studies have been conducted in this area that do help guide decision making.

If we look at everyone who has had a first unprovoked seizure, the overall risk of recurrence is a little less than 50 percent. In other words, a little more than half of these people will *not* go on to have further seizures. However, some important information is lost when we look at everyone together. If you have had a single seizure, there are some factors that can help your doctor individualize *your* risk of having another seizure. These factors include the underlying cause of the seizure (if known), the timing of the seizure (nighttime seizures have higher risk of recurrence), and abnormal findings on EEG or MRI. While there is no single test to predict this risk, we can add up these important factors. Your doctor will consider your seizure type and any findings on your neurologic examination and tests to help determine your individual risk of seizure recurrence.

Most often, your doctor will not recommend treatment after a single seizure unless predictors of a higher risk of recurrence are identified. Matt had none of the factors that predicted a higher chance of seizure recurrence. From study of many other people in similar circumstances, we know that his chances of having more seizures is about 30 percent. Looking at it from the other direction, the chances that he would *not* have another seizure was about 70 percent. Matt and his doctor, like most people in this situation, decided against daily AED therapy. Matt plans to be very careful to stay with limited, moderate alcohol use and to avoid sleep deprivation whenever possible.

When an approximate risk of seizure recurrence can be estimated, it can help promote a discussion between you and your doctor to find the best choice for you. Not everyone with the same risk of recurrence will make the same decision. For example, consider the situation where there is an approximately 50 percent chance of seizure recurrence. The decision making may be very different for a college student who does not drive, a soccer mom who is driving her three children to different activities all day (see Chapter 3 on driving), and different still for a young woman who is planning on starting a family and who may want to avoid the risk of birth defects from AEDs (see Chapter 13 on AEDs and women's health). Efforts to promote safety and prevent seizures have to be weighed against concerns about medication cost and possible exposure to medication side effects. The decision to start daily medication can also change your view of your health. Instead of a single seizure that doesn't require treatment, it now seems more like a medical condition that needs daily therapy.

Nonpharmacological Approaches to Reducing Seizure Risk

In the previous section we saw how part of Matt's plan going forward was a commitment to limiting alcohol use and getting adequate sleep.

Once a decision has been made to treat, there is a temptation to jump right to talking about the various AED options and to rely exclusively on medication to manage seizures. In doing so, there is a risk of skipping past a discussion of other useful approaches. As a group, these approaches involve lifestyle management to eliminate factors that might generally lower the threshold for having seizures or specifically trigger seizures in some individuals. Other more specific non-AED approaches, such as medical devices, epilepsy surgery, and nonconventional and diet therapies, will be discussed in Chapter 12.

Can people with epilepsy identify factors that trigger their seizures? For many, the answer is a resounding yes! Some studies of people with epilepsy have suggested that up to 90 percent of people with epilepsy are able to identify triggers for their seizures. In most cases, there does indeed seem to be a biological link to explain the trigger. Of course, we must always be aware of the human tendency to find explanations where there are none and incorrectly connect seizures with an unrelated event; however, this appears to be less common (Box 8–1).

> **BOX 8-1 Common Seizure Triggers**
>
> - Stress
> - Sleep deprivation
> - Alcohol and drug use, including certain prescription drugs
> - Illness or fever
> - Forgetting to take seizure medications
> - Menses (in some women)
> - Specific triggers, such as flashing lights

Stress Reduction

The most commonly cited trigger for seizures is stress. In most cases the connection is with psychological or emotional stresses, although physical stress or exhaustion is also reported by some to be a trigger. This is an area that has been notoriously hard to study. Stress is hard to measure. Perhaps it is even harder to avoid! Nonetheless, because stress comes up so consistently as a trigger, it is likely a meaningful one. It is difficult, if not impossible, to eliminate all stress from one's life. Many of the approaches to raising awareness of and managing stress fall outside of conventional medicine and often into the realm of complementary and alternative medicine (CAM). Read on to find out more about stress reduction approaches in Chapter 12.

Avoiding Sleep Deprivation

Sleep deprivation and fatigue are also commonly reported triggers. In fact, when we are trying to bring out EEG abnormalities in the lab or record seizures during video-EEG monitoring in the epilepsy monitoring unit, we often ask patients to stay awake much of the night and become sleep deprived. Many studies have shown that sleep deprivation will produce more spikes and sharp waves on EEG. For many people, it will also increase the chances of having a seizure. This especially appears to be the case for people who have a generalized epilepsy syndrome with a genetic cause. Examples of these include juvenile myoclonic epilepsy, juvenile absence epilepsy, and epilepsy with generalized tonic-clonic seizures alone. However, people with many different epilepsy syndromes are potentially vulnerable to the effects of sleep deprivation.

Sleep problems are very common and are seen even more often in people with epilepsy. Taking sleeping pills for long periods of time is usually not a good solution. A good starting point is to talk with your primary care provider or neurologist. Often developing some good basic sleep habits can go a long way to improving things.

Should you worry if you don't get a good night's sleep on one occasion? No. Should you avoid extremes of sleep deprivation? Yes. Should you follow treatment for sleep disorders such as sleep apnea if you have it? Yes. These measures can help make medications work better.

Managing Alcohol and Drug Use

What about alcohol and drugs? Both can lower the seizure threshold and serve as triggers for seizures. In extreme circumstances, alcohol and drug use can provoke seizures in people who aren't otherwise prone to seizures. In people who *do* have epilepsy, the same factors can be at work, but it is likely that less extreme circumstances may be required to trigger a seizure. Let's be a little more specific.

Alcohol can clearly make seizures more likely to occur. Getting drunk or "buzzed" can trigger seizures. Your risk of seizures will be increased the next day also, as the effects of the alcohol wear off. Alcohol can also combine in bad ways with antiepileptic medications to multiply the side effects of these drugs. Some people with epilepsy choose to cut out alcohol altogether. Many others find that they are able to have an occasional glass of wine or beer with dinner and not have problems with seizures or medication side effects. It is important to talk with your doctor to find out what is best for you.

It is very important for people with a history of seizures to avoid drugs of abuse that are stimulants. These include cocaine and methamphetamine. Stimulant drugs can have many bad health effects, including triggering seizures. I have several patients whose seizures have been triggered by "energy drinks," and these are probably best avoided also. Low to moderate caffeine use (for example, a cup of coffee each morning) is well tolerated by most people.

Avoiding Drug Withdrawal

Equally problematic can be withdrawal from certain medications. Problems are seen most often with medications in the class called benzodiazepines, which include diazepam (Valium) or clonazepam (Klonopin). These medications are often used to treat anxiety but also commonly to treat epilepsy. When people take benzodiazepines for a long time, the body and brain become used to them, and stopping them suddenly can trigger seizures. Withdrawal seizures from benzodiazepines can happen in people with epilepsy or even in people who do not have epilepsy and are not otherwise prone to having seizures. The process of alcohol withdrawal seizures is similar—steady, excessive daily use followed by suddenly stopping use can cause problems, including seizures.

Avoiding Strobe Lights

For some people with epilepsy, flashing lights (photic stimulation) needs to be avoided. Some of you may recall the story of the infamous *Pokémon* episode. In December 1997, when the Japanese cartoon *Pokémon* was near the height of its popularity, an episode was aired on Japanese television that had an estimated viewing audience of 10 million, including an estimated 55 percent of all school-age children in Japan. This particular episode contained a scene with rapidly flashing images with color changes. As a consequence, 685 children in Japan had seizures. Half of them had no previous history of seizures, and about one-third required hospitalization overnight. This led to stricter guidelines that limit rapid flashing and color changes in television, movies, and videogames. Sensitivity to flashing lights, or "photosensitivity," is seen most frequently in people with genetic generalized epilepsies, such as juvenile myoclonic epilepsy. Flashing lights are the most common specific trigger for seizures, but is seen in only about 5 percent of people with epilepsy. Most seizures have no identified trigger. Photosensitivity is more common in girls or women than boys and men.

People with photosensitive epilepsy should avoid rapidly flashing lights. For some people, the flicker seen in old cathode ray tube (CRT) screens can cause problems. Fortunately, this is not the case with newer flat-panel (LCD) screens. Risk can also be minimized by viewing content in a well-lit room and sitting well back from the screen. If suddenly exposed to flashing lights, the risk of having a seizure is greatly reduced by simply closing one eye.

Flashing lights are the most common specific trigger for seizures; rarely, however, there can be other very specific triggers for seizures. As a group these are called "reflex" epilepsies. In people with reflex epilepsies, seizures are triggered mostly or exclusively by external or internal stimuli. They are rare, but there is an amazing variety of different specific triggers. External triggers include touch or startle, specific visual patterns, specific sounds or pieces of music, hot water, or food. Internal triggers can include certain patterns of thought, including mental calculations, reading, and playing chess. I have had several patients with startle-induced seizures, where unexpected daily encounters such as a ringing telephone or an unexpected snap from stepping on a dry twig can trigger seizures and falls.

You can see that a wide variety of actions and behaviors can lower the threshold for or trigger seizures. Some are easily avoided, some can be modified with some effort, and others are simply unavoidable.

It is worth thinking through these general and specific factors to see what might be influencing seizures for you or your friend or family member. Rarely is avoidance of triggers alone adequate to control seizures. But minimizing these risks can go a long way toward achieving the goal of complete control of seizures with no side effects.

Stopping AEDs

You might be concerned about long-term side effects of AEDs. After months or years with no seizures, you might wonder if they are still needed. Once started, can AEDs ever be stopped? The answer for teens and adults is a limited yes.

Your doctor will use some information to help answer this question for you. If your doctor knows your epilepsy syndrome, that can provide a lot of guidance. A few childhood-onset epilepsy syndromes, such as childhood absence epilepsy, are age dependent. This means that they typically appear at a certain stage of development and then are "outgrown" at a certain age. For childhood absence epilepsy that age is usually adolescence. It is very rare for an adult to require continued treatment for childhood absence epilepsy.

For epilepsy that begins in adolescence or adulthood, the outlook for stopping AEDs is often less clear and less optimistic. One common type of epilepsy that starts in teenage years is called juvenile myoclonic epilepsy (JME). JME can often be effectively treated with AED therapy, but it is rarely "outgrown"; lifelong therapy is more the rule, and stopping AEDs the exception, for this epilepsy syndrome.

Most people with adult-onset epilepsy have focal-onset seizures and one of the focal epilepsy syndromes. If known, the cause of the epilepsy may help predict whether AEDs can be safely discontinued at some point. Often there is not a simple answer and no single test that can be done to determine if someone can safely stop AED therapy. However, your doctor can use some basic principles to guide decision making.

In most cases, a person must be free of seizures for at least 2 years before stopping AEDs is considered. Your doctor may order a repeat EEG to help with decision making. If clear abnormalities are seen on the EEG, your doctor will likely advise that you stay on AED therapy to prevent seizures. A normal EEG is good, but EEG is not a perfect test. Some people with normal EEGs may still have recurrent seizures after stopping AEDs. A normal EEG is not a "clean bill of health." Your doctor will consider other factors beyond the EEG that are at least equally important. Favorable factors include:

- Control of seizures is achieved easily on one drug at a low dose
- There have been no previous unsuccessful attempts at withdrawal
- The neurologic examination, MRI, and EEG are all normal
- Seizures are primary generalized (rather than focal onset)— except for the syndrome of JME

If many of these features are met and you have been seizure free for more than 2 years, gradual AED discontinuation may be considered.

In many ways, the decision about whether to stop AEDs is the mirror image of the decision of whether to *start* AED therapy. In both cases, the decision must be individualized. Faced with the same risk of recurrence after stopping AEDs, you might make a different decision from your neighbor. If you are a woman who has been seizure free for 5 years and who is planning a future pregnancy, you might be very motivated to attempt a taper to avoid the risks of AEDs during pregnancy. If you drive a truck for a living, you might make a very different decision. The consequences of a possible breakthrough seizure when AEDs are stopped, including on driving and work, must be carefully considered.

Chapter 9

Antiepileptic Drug Therapy

This chapter is central to understanding treatment of epilepsy. When treatment is needed, it almost always begins with antiepileptic medications. In this chapter we will briefly look at how these medications work, discuss some basic principles of treatment with antiepileptic medications, and then devote the rest of the chapter to talking about how your doctor will select the correct medication for you.

Marta did not expect to develop epilepsy. No one in her family was known to have seizures, nor had she ever experienced a seizure as a child. But at age 31, she found herself in the emergency department after a generalized tonic-clonic seizure. She had been on the bus going home when she experienced an intense feeling in her stomach that moved in a warm rush up to her chest and head. It was very difficult to describe, but it was a little like the feeling of dropping on a roller coaster or moving in a fast elevator. That was all she could recall, but others on the bus said she moaned, stiffened, and convulsed for about a minute. Her blood tests and CT scan of the brain in the emergency department were normal.

The emergency department staff asked careful questions about any other similar episodes. She was certain that she had never had a convulsion before. However, she admitted that she *had* experienced the roller coaster feeling before, just never quite this intensely. It had happened three times in the

(Continued)

(Continued)
past 2 months, and the second time she felt a little confused afterward and had to pause to remember where she was and what she was doing. Marta is a certified public accountant (CPA), it was tax season, and she assumed she had just been working too hard.

The physician in the emergency department recognized that the convulsion was not her first but in fact her *fourth* seizure. She had experienced two simple partial seizures (auras) and probably a brief complex partial seizure previously (when she felt confused and had trouble recalling where she was). He felt she had epilepsy and gave Marta an intravenous form of a medication called phenytoin (Dilantin) so that she would be rapidly protected from further seizures, as well as a prescription for phenytoin capsules to take at home.

We can use Marta's experience as a jumping-off point to talk about antiepileptic drugs. Remember: AEDs are generally not used to treat people with *provoked* seizures. Most people with a single seizure are not treated with AEDs unless the risk of recurrence is felt to be high. Nearly all people with repeated, unprovoked seizures (epilepsy) require treatment. But how does a doctor know what medication is the right one to use?

AED Mechanisms

We will delay the discussion of AED choice for a moment while we briefly talk about AED mechanisms (how they work) and explore how much of a role this plays in AED choice.

In Chapter 4 we reviewed some of the basic mechanisms by which seizures are produced. We saw that seizures result from an imbalance in the brain between excitation (the gas pedal—too much) and inhibition (the brake pedal—too little). This imbalance can sometimes be explained by problems with charged particles like sodium, potassium, and calcium, or the channels that control their flow. At other times the electrical or chemical signaling systems that direct this fine balance could be disrupted—too many excitatory or too few inhibitory signals. Having this understanding about seizure mechanisms can go a long way toward explaining how AEDs are developed and why they work.

Without going into too much detail about the chemistry, we can see how AEDs target some of these basic mechanisms and how knowledge of the mechanisms might guide AED selection, especially when used in combination (polytherapy).

One of the early events in the firing of a brain cell (called an **action potential**) involves channels for sodium rapidly opening. Not surprisingly many AEDs act by blocking the opening of sodium channels. Blocking calcium channels can have a similar effect, and this is a mechanism employed by some AEDs. Opening of some channels (for example, potassium or chloride) makes it *more difficult* for the brain cell to fire, and AEDs that open potassium and chloride channels both exist. Other drugs target the chemical messengers (**neurotransmitters**) that control these channels. In theory, one could block excitatory neurotransmitters (those that promote cell firing), or boost inhibitory neurotransmitters (those that reduce cell firing). In practice, both of these systems exist. The main excitatory neurotransmitter in the brain is called **glutamate**. When glutamate is released, it attaches to a receptor on another cell and makes that cell more likely to fire. Several AEDs use blocking of the glutamate receptor as a mechanism. The main inhibitory neurotransmitter in the brain is called gamma-aminobutyric acid, or **GABA**. Many drugs seek to boost GABA levels in the brain and thus make seizures less likely to occur.

The details of these mechanisms are more important for the health professional who is prescribing your medication and for the scientists busy at work developing new drugs. However, understanding these mechanisms is also very important for selecting the right seizure medication for an individual. If the epilepsy syndrome is known, then perhaps a medication with a specific mechanism to treat that syndrome could be targeted. If more than one medication is needed, perhaps doctors could choose medications with mechanisms that work well together.

In practice, the ability to predict effectiveness of medication combinations on the basis of mechanism is less fully developed than one might guess. For a given epilepsy syndrome, several drugs with different mechanisms of action could be chosen. When selecting two drugs that might work well together (polytherapy), a drug's mechanism is taken into consideration. Usually there is some effort to avoid choosing drugs with the same mechanism, as those combinations might be less effective and more likely to produce side effects.

However, the science has not advanced enough to use mechanism of action as the primary factor for identifying ideal medication combinations. While this idea is appealing, the best combinations are not always predictable for an individual person, and a fair amount of trial and error is still involved. In the future, as we continue to learn more about mechanisms and how they interact with a specific person's unique biology, this may change.

Basic Principles of AED Therapy

Before we discuss AED choice, let's review the guiding principles. What is the goal of AED therapy? In fact, there are two main goals: to stop the seizures and to not cause any new problems in the process. In short, no seizures, no side effects. Becoming seizure free can remove many practical restrictions on driving and other activities. It clearly leads to improved sense of well-being and quality of life. In children, avoiding seizures can help permit normal brain development and learning. And finally, getting rapid and complete seizure control can avoid many of the long-term problems associated with poorly controlled seizures.

The Range of AED Choices

Following the development of phenobarbital as an antiepileptic medication in 1912, new medications were gradually added over the next 80 or so years. However, the 1990s saw the beginning of an outpouring of new medications to treat epilepsy. Some of these advances resulted from the work of the National Institutes of Health (NIH)/National Institute of Neurological Disorders and Stroke (NINDS) Anticonvulsant Screening Program, some were developed by the pharmaceutical industry, and some from a collaboration among industry, independent scientists, and government. Figure 9–1 shows the date of introduction of some of the more commonly used AEDs and emphasizes the point that available medication options have more than doubled over the past 25 years. This

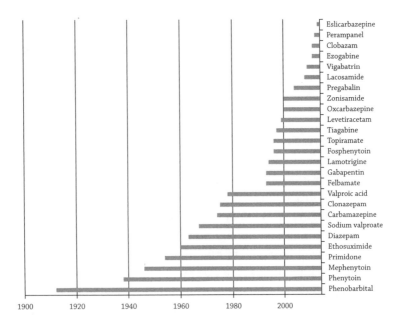

FIGURE 9-1 Timeline of AED development.

has provided a wonderful range of options for treatment, but the sheer number of medications to select from is daunting.

AED Selection

To look at AED selection, we will break down the process in two different ways.

First, your doctor needs to understand what type of epilepsy you have so that the best treatment can be selected. If testing has allowed identification of your specific epilepsy syndrome, that can be very helpful. Short of that, the most important distinction is between *focal-onset* and *generalized-onset* seizures, which are treated differently; we will examine them separately. Within these groups some of the differences are less important. For example, if you have focal seizures, differences in *location* of seizure onset are less meaningful. A focal seizure coming from the temporal lobe is treated much the same as a focal seizure coming from the frontal lobe. Differences in the specific *cause* of your epilepsy are also of secondary importance; focal seizures caused by head trauma or by a stroke respond to similar treatments.

Second, we will differentiate older and newer medications and discuss when and why your doctor might choose one over the other.

As you can see in Figure 9–2, your doctor needs to know the epilepsy syndrome—or at least whether you have focal or generalized-onset seizures—as a central factor in AED selection. Then, there are multiple other factors that your doctor must consider when deciding which AED will be best for you. The process includes (a) generating a list of possible options, (b) narrowing the list based on the considerations listed in Figure 9–2, and (c) making a selection.

Often the AEDs don't appear very different from one another in effectiveness. There are some differences in effectiveness between various AEDs, but these are sometimes subtle or hard to predict for a specific individual. More often a doctor will select an AED based

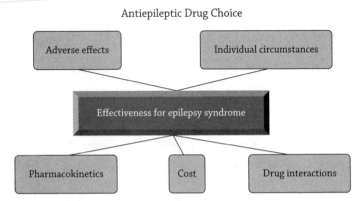

FIGURE 9-2 Factors affecting AED choice.

on the other surrounding factors. The ideal AED for an individual is one that has a low likelihood of causing side effects and will not make worse (and possibly could help) other existing medical conditions. Ideally it would also be simple to use, require infrequent dosing, would not interact with other medications, and would be inexpensive. It is in these other factors that some of the bigger differences between AEDs are seen and therefore are very important in guiding your doctor's choice of the best medication for you from the list of possible options (Table 9–1).

AED Selection in Focal Epilepsy

Let's begin with AED selection in focal epilepsies. It is worth repeating that in addition to simple partial and complex partial seizures, secondarily generalized tonic-clonic seizures fall into this category. Thus someone who has generalized tonic-clonic seizures (formerly called "grand mal" seizures) may often have a *focal-onset* epilepsy (they are *secondarily* generalized) and therefore are part of this discussion.

TABLE 9-1 Antiepileptic Drugs in Common Use

Drug	Brand Names
phenobarbital	Phenobarbital
phenytoin	Dilantin, Phenytek
primidone	Mysoline
ethosuximide	Zarontin
diazepam	Valium
diazepam (rectal)	Diastat
sodium valproate	Depakote
sodium valproate (extended release)	Depakote ER
sodium valproate (intravenous)	Depacon
carbamazepine	Tegretol
carbamazepine (extended release)	Carbatrol, Tegretol XR
clonazepam	Klonopin
lorazepam	Ativan
valproic acid	Depakene
felbamate	Felbatol
gabapentin	Neurontin
lamotrigine	Lamictal
lamotrigine (extended release)	Lamictal XR
fosphenytoin	Phenytek
topiramate	Topamax
topiramate (extended release)	Trokendi XR, Qudexy XR
tiagabine	Gabitril
levetiracetam	Keppra
levetiracetam (extended release)	Keppra XR
oxcarbazepine	Trileptal
oxcarbazepine (extended release)	Oxtellar XR
zonisamide	Zonegran
pregabalin	Lyrica
lacosamide	Vimpat
rufinamide	Banzel
vigabatrin	Sabril
ezogabine	Potiga
clobazam	Onfi
perampanel	Fycompa
eslicarbazepine	Aptiom

Older AEDs

We introduced the section on AED therapy with the story of Marta, who had a seizure on the bus and who was newly diagnosed with epilepsy in the emergency department. We discovered that she has focal epilepsy and had experienced simple partial, complex partial, and secondarily generalized seizures. What is the best way to choose a medication for Marta?

Let's start by briefly taking a ride in a time machine back to the 1980s. Remember big hair? Michael Jackson and Madonna? *Cheers* and *The Cosby Show*? It was a simpler time for AED treatment because the choices were more limited and some good comparative data helped to guide choices.

For focal-onset seizures, the main options included a barbiturate (phenobarbital or primidone [Mysoline], a drug that is converted into phenobarbital), phenytoin (Dilantin), carbamazepine (Tegretol), or sodium valproate/valproic acid (Depakote/Depakene).

A series of comparisons of these drugs was made, and an interesting finding emerged. The barbiturates (phenobarbital, primidone) were as effective for controlling seizures as the others but were less well tolerated (more side effects), so they were less preferred. Sodium valproate (Depakote) seemed to control secondarily generalized seizures well, but was slightly less effective in stopping complex partial seizures, so was less preferred.

Thus in that era, phenytoin (Dilantin) and carbamazepine (Tegretol) emerged as the "drugs of choice" for treating focal-onset seizures. They were equally effective in controlling seizures and about equally well tolerated. Often carbamazepine (Tegretol) was considered first choice because it lacked some of the long-term side effects that could be seen with phenytoin (Dilantin), such as excessive hair growth, coarsening of facial features, and overgrowth of the gums.

A lot has changed since the 1980s, and not just the hairstyles and music. A large number of newer antiepileptic medications have since become available and are now in widespread use. These are too numerous to practically review each one individually here, but you will find a listing, along with some of the more notable features of each drug, in Appendix 2. Here we will focus on some general principles.

Newer AEDs

The first important point about the newer AEDs is that *they are not necessarily more effective* in stopping seizures than the older drugs. This may seem surprising given all of the time, effort, and brainpower that has gone into developing new AEDs. But if you compare a study from the 1980s to a current study, the findings are amazingly similar: In both cases about one-third of patients don't achieve complete seizure control with AED therapy (old or new). Why then would there be an advantage to using newer medications?

Most of the advantages of the newer drugs are in other areas. Some of the newer AEDs show better tolerability than older AEDs. They may produce fewer short- and long-term side effects. This is extremely important for drugs that have to be taken daily, often for years. Many of the newer drugs are also processed by the body (metabolized) in simpler ways. As we will see, this can make it easier to maintain steady blood levels and can also help to avoid medication interactions—both with other drugs that are being taken and with other AEDs. Some newer AEDs are long lasting in the body or have extended-release forms, allowing for less frequent dosing. Some of the newer drugs may be better suited to certain people with other health issues. If you have liver disease, you might benefit from a medication that is not processed by the liver but simply cleared by the kidneys. If you are overweight, you might doubly benefit from using an AED that controls seizures *and* promotes weight loss. We will see that these differences from the older medications can make a big difference for many people, particularly in some special populations.

Where to Begin?

Before we talk about *which* medication, let's talk about *how many*. If you have a new diagnosis of epilepsy, the choice is very clear: single-drug therapy (**monotherapy**) is best. In the distant past the recommendation was sometimes made to start two AEDs together (**polytherapy**) at the time of diagnosis. Here are some of the disadvantages of this approach:

Potential Disadvantages of Polytherapy

- Increased side effects
- Greater chances of toxicity
- Difficult-to-manage drug interactions
- Less success in remembering to take medications correctly
- Higher cost
- Increased chances of causing birth defects in women with epilepsy

Ultimately, the most important reason is that monotherapy is sufficient for most people. It is recommended to investigate monotherapy fully before adding a second drug.

How successful is monotherapy? Several studies have looked at this issue and can provide some approximate numbers. In general, about half of the people started on a first monotherapy trial gain complete control of seizures without problematic side effects. Another 10 to 15 percent got complete seizure control without important side effects with a second monotherapy trial. If the first trial failed because of side effects (not for lack of effectiveness), the chances that the second trial will be successful are even higher. Further monotherapy and polytherapy trials can definitely improve seizure control and minimize side effects. But only a small additional number of people go on to achieve the goal: complete seizure control. Therefore we think we can identify early those people who are destined to have medication-resistant epilepsy. Not every available medication must be tried before identifying a medication-resistant form of epilepsy. This is very important because many of those people might be good candidates for epilepsy surgery or other non-AED therapy. Early identification of these individuals can allow this process to move forward before years or decades of poor seizure control take their toll.

Options for Monotherapy with Newer AEDs in Focal Epilepsy

The list of newer AEDs that are active against focal epilepsy is long (Table 9–2). For simplicity, I have removed some of the duplicate extended-release forms from the list. Which of these can be used as

TABLE 9-2 Newer AEDs That Are Active against Focal Epilepsy

Drug	Brand
felbamate*	Felbatol
gabapentin	Neurontin
lamotrigine*	Lamictal
topiramate*	Topamax
tiagabine	Gabitril
levetiracetam	Keppra
oxcarbazepine*	Trileptal
zonisamide	Zonegran
pregabalin	Lyrica
lacosamide	Vimpat
vigabatrin	Sabril
ezogabine	Potiga
perampanel	Fycompa
eslicarbazepine	Aptiom

single-drug therapy? The answer is a little more complicated than you might think.

Most AEDs for partial epilepsy are first studied and approved as add-on or adjunctive therapy. For a drug to be approved as monotherapy, an additional set of time-consuming and expensive studies are required. Several in Table 9–2 (marked by the *) have gone through this process and have official US Food and Drug Administration (FDA) approval for use as monotherapy. This gives greater assurance that these medications work not only as add-on therapy, but that they are also adequate for use as monotherapy.

Does this mean that the many drugs not marked with a star are *not* effective as monotherapy? Definitely not. Since they work as adjunctive therapy, there is every reason to expect that they might also work as monotherapy, but often the additional studies to prove this have not been done. Some of these drugs are commonly used as monotherapy, even though they don't have official approval to be used in this way. When this is done, it is said that the drug is being used **off-label**.

When choosing among the newer AEDs for focal epilepsy, neurologists have access to a few studies comparing drugs that can be used to help make the best choice. The main message from these studies is that it is difficult to show big differences in effectiveness between the different drugs. However, the newer AEDs are often superior to the older drugs in tolerability. More people taking the newer AEDs are able to stay on effective therapy because they feel better—they don't have daily side effects that cause them to stop therapy.

There is still much we don't know about AEDs, but here are some of the main take-home messages that neurologists consider when trying to determine which drug to prescribe:

- The goal is to be seizure free without side effects
- Treatment should start with monotherapy
- Many AED options are available for the treatment of focal-onset epilepsy

- Older AEDs can be effective for treating seizures but may have some disadvantages compared with newer drugs, especially for certain groups of people, such as older patients or women
- As a group, newer AEDs are not clearly more effective than older AEDs, but:
  - They offer a greater range of choices
  - A newer AED may be more effective for a specific individual
  - Many newer AEDs have better tolerability and thus may be more "successful" overall for treating the epilepsy
  - Many newer AEDs have fewer drug–drug interactions
- The course of treatment should be reconsidered if seizure control without side effects is not achieved after the first two to three AED trials

Failure of Monotherapy in Focal Epilepsy

When might your neurologist need to switch from monotherapy to polytherapy? There is no single correct answer and limited scientific evidence to guide this decision. Epilepsy experts differ in their answer to this question and their approach to treatment. Commonly, your neurologist might explore two monotherapy trials thoroughly before moving on to polytherapy.

Not everyone whose seizures fail to respond to early AED trials simply has drug-resistant epilepsy. If there is not a good response to initial trials, your neurologist should be considering the following possibilities:

- The diagnosis is incorrect (trying to treat a nonepilepsy condition with AEDs).
- An underlying progressive neurologic disorder is present that is making treatment difficult (for example, a growing brain tumor).

- The choice of AED was incorrect for the epilepsy syndrome.
- The dose of the AED was too low to stop the seizures.
- Side effects of the particular medication(s) chosen limit the ability to get to an effective dose.
- There are drug–drug interactions that are making the AED less effective.
- For various reasons, the AED is being irregularly dosed, leading to incomplete seizure control from low AED levels.
- Some other factor, such as ongoing alcohol or substance use, is making the AED less effective.

Thus many possible options exist to improve seizure control when initial monotherapy fails. You can help your neurologist in this process by being as accurate and open as possible about factors that might affect your seizure control.

AED Selection in Generalized Epilepsy

Remember at the start of this section that we split epilepsy syndromes into those that are focal in onset (just discussed) and those that are generalized in onset (discussed here). Recall from Chapter 2 that the generalized-from-onset seizure types include the following:

- Absence seizures
- Atypical absence seizures
- Myoclonic seizures
- (Generalized-from-onset) Generalized tonic-clonic seizures
- Atonic seizures
- Tonic seizures

Within the group of people who have generalized-from-onset seizures, some may have specific epilepsy syndromes that can be determined from typical medical histories, patterns of seizure types, and results of testing. Other times this kind of specificity is not possible, and we may classify the seizures just in the broad category of a generalized epilepsy syndrome.

If you have been diagnosed with a form of generalized epilepsy, your neurologist may likely prescribe an AED from the following, more limited list:

- Sodium valproate (Depakote)
- Lamotrigine (Lamictal)
- Ethosuximide (Zarontin)
- Topiramate (Topamax)
- Levetiracetam (Keppra)
- Zonisamide (Zonegran)
- Felbamate (Felbatol)
- Rufinamide (Banzel)
- Clobazam (Onfi)
- Other benzodiazepines (for example, clonazepam [Klonopin] or clorazepate [Tranxene])

Some of these medications (for example, topiramate and levetiracetam) you may recognize from the list of drugs for focal epilepsy. The medications that appear on both lists are often considered to be **broad-spectrum AEDs**. Broad-spectrum AEDs are generally effective treatments for people with either focal or generalized epilepsy, which raises the first and one of the most important principles of treating generalized-from-onset seizures:

- If you have a form of generalized epilepsy, a medication that is specific for focal epilepsy (**narrow-spectrum AED**) could make your seizures worse.

Use of drugs that specifically treat focal epilepsy (such as carbamazepine, oxcarbazepine, or gabapentin) in someone with generalized-from-onset seizures may not be effective for control of the seizures. In fact, at times it can make the seizures *worse*. While there are always exceptions to the rule, more often than not this principle holds.

Mostly we'll discuss principles that apply to everyone in this group, regardless of syndrome, but some additional comments will be made that apply to two subgroups:

- Genetic generalized epilepsies
- Symptomatic generalized epilepsies

For the most part, people with genetic generalized epilepsies don't have other neurologic problems besides their seizures. Their tendency to have generalized seizures is on a genetic basis, sometimes inherited (passed down from other family members), and at other times just occurring in that individual. Examples include the syndromes of childhood absence epilepsy, juvenile absence epilepsy, juvenile myoclonic epilepsy (JME), and epilepsy with generalized tonic-clonic seizures alone.

People with symptomatic generalized epilepsies often have generalized seizures as a "symptom" of another neurologic process going on. The epilepsy usually begins in childhood, and can then continue into adolescence and adulthood. The cause may be different in different people but often is a process that involves a large part of the brain or multiple areas of both sides of the brain. Examples of these causes might include brain malformations, lack of oxygen at birth, infections, trauma, or chromosomal abnormalities. A number of specific syndromes in this group are seen in childhood, but the most common one to continue into adolescence and adulthood is called **Lennox-Gastaut syndrome (LGS)**. People with this epilepsy syndrome often have some degree of intellectual disability, a certain pattern on their EEG called slow spike and wave, and often several types of generalized-from-onset seizures. However, not all of these features are needed to establish the syndrome diagnosis.

Older AEDs for Generalized Epilepsy

In our discussion of medications for focal epilepsy, we began by talking about older AEDs. If we took our time machine for another spin back to the 1980s we would find a limited number of options. Sodium valproate (Depakote) would be widely acknowledged as the drug of choice for many of the generalized-from-onset seizures. Ethosuximide (Zarontin) would be used in children who had only **absence seizures**. And different medications in the class of benzodiazepines (for example, clonazepam [Klonopin]) might also be fairly widely used.

While sodium valproate was recognized as being very effective for generalized-from-onset seizures, it also has a number of potential side effects (discussed in Chapter 10 and in Appendix 2). Because of this, the development of new options for treating generalized-from-onset seizures with newer medications was welcomed.

Newer AEDs for Generalized Epilepsy

Let's look a little more carefully at the list of drugs commonly used for generalized-from-onset seizures listed at the start of this section. These drugs are generally considered broad spectrum and appropriate for use in people with generalized epilepsy. Newer AEDs that are commonly used for the treatment of generalized epilepsy include lamotrigine, topiramate, levetiracetam, zonisamide, clobazam, and other medications in the class called benzodiazepines.

Some of the medications on the list are used less often or more narrowly in specific groups of people.

Felbamate (Felbatol) was found to have very serious side effects in some people—liver or bone marrow failure leading to death—and thus is not a first-choice medication. It is only used in a small number of people in whom the potential benefit is felt to outweigh the known risks.

Ethosuximide (Zarontin) is used mostly in children and infrequently in adults. It is mostly used for a syndrome called childhood absence epilepsy. It acts specifically to control absence seizures but is not effective against generalized tonic-clonic seizures, which may also be seen in people with absence seizures. Thus if someone has both of these seizure types, ethosuximide alone is not adequate. Another drug must be used with it, or a drug that covers both seizure types (many of the others on this list), must be used.

Lamotrigine (Lamictal), topiramate (Topamax), levetiracetam (Keppra) and zonisamide (Zonegran) are considered by most epilepsy experts to be relatively broad-spectrum AEDs. They are used to treat focal-onset seizures, but also are effective in treating generalized-onset seizures.

The two remaining drugs (rufinamide [Banzel] and clobazam [Onfi]) entered the market most recently with approval for a specific syndrome, Lennox-Gastaut syndrome. LGS is a specific symptomatic generalized epilepsy syndrome that is often severe and in which multiple different generalized seizure types are seen. Rufinamide and clobazam have been used off-label, for example in other symptomatic generalized epilepsies.

As with focal epilepsy, a few studies have been conducted comparing drugs for generalized-from-onset epilepsies to help determine which should be first-choice options. These studies showed that some of the older drugs, like sodium valproate (Depakote), were the most effective.

If you have generalized epilepsy, does that mean that your neurologist should choose an older drug for you? No, it is not that simple. Your neurologist will consider many other factors. Sometimes the differences in the effectiveness of different medications are very small and may be overshadowed by factors such as the possible side effects of drugs. Let's consider Emily, for example.

Emily, who was 17 years old, was diagnosed with juvenile myoclonic epilepsy (JME) after she had two generalized tonic-clonic seizures when sleep deprived. She also had a history

(Continued)

(*Continued*)

of myoclonic seizures that started several months before the generalized tonic-clonic seizures. She and her neurologist discussed that sodium valproate might likely have a slight edge in effectiveness compared to other AED options. However, they also discussed the common side effects of sodium valproate: weight gain, tremor, and sometimes hair loss. Sodium valproate also has the highest rate of causing birth defects of all the AEDs. Emily was not planning to start a family in the immediate future, but she would probably need lifelong treatment for her epilepsy, and the issue was likely to come up at some point. After this discussion, Emily and her doctor agreed that she could start by trying an alternative. If the alternatives did not adequately control seizures, sodium valproate could be reconsidered.

An Approach to AED Selection

You have probably gotten the sense from the preceding discussion that it would be difficult to come up with a single recipe for making the best AED choice for everyone. But I hope that the discussion has also revealed some of the principles that neurologists consider in helping guide AED selection:

- They will work to understand as much about the seizure type(s) and epilepsy syndrome as possible.
- For focal-onset seizures and localized epilepsy syndromes, they will choose among the many medications that are effective for focal or partial-onset seizures.
- For generalized-from-onset seizures, they will select from the smaller group of medications that are appropriate for those seizure types.

- If the epilepsy syndrome is not known with certainty, they will select a broad-spectrum AED that might be effective for either focal or generalized-onset seizures.
- Tolerability and potential side effects, among other factors, may guide many of the choices that are made—more so than differences in effectiveness.
- After all of the evidence for the best AED choice is considered, the process of coming to a good final decision includes experience, judgment, and teamwork between provider and patient.

Debates in Epilepsy: Generic versus Brand Name AEDs

Substitution of generic for brand name medications is a controversial area in epilepsy care. To explore this issue, let's think about a common issue that arose with my patient Jerry, who was 58 years old and had had well-controlled epilepsy for many years on the brand name form of his AED in monotherapy. Jerry received notice from his insurance company stating that he would need to make a $200-per-month copay if he wished to continue his brand name medication. Alternatively, he could "choose" to switch to the generic form of the AED for a $10-per-month copay. Jerry was uncertain about what was the right thing to do. He was reluctant to change because he had been seizure free on the brand name AED, and he had heard concerns that generic medications were not as good. On the other hand, maybe the generic would be no different, and he would save a lot of money.

(Continued)

(Continued)

Would Jerry be putting himself at risk by taking a generic medication? Wherever there is controversy, it is good to begin with some facts.

The first fact is that use of generic medications has sky-rocketed over the last couple of decades. Generic medications now make up well over half of prescribed medications in the United States and a majority of prescribed AEDs. What rules govern generic AED equivalents?

Generic drugs are regulated by the FDA. The rigorous manufacturing and packaging standards are the same as for brand name drugs. They must contain the same active drug in the same strength, within strict limits. Small variation is permitted, but a recent study of a large number of generic preparations showed that the difference between brand name and generics was very small and averaged about 3.5 percent. Even brand name medications may also show some variation between different batches or "lots" of medication that are manufactured.

How do these facts relate to AED use? There are arguments both for and against the use of generic AEDs. The main argument *for* generic use is cost. The United States has the highest per-person drug costs in the world, and, on average, generic drugs cost about 80 percent less than their brand name equivalents.

The arguments against generic substitution are several. First, generic drugs are demonstrated to be "equivalent" to brand name drugs in short studies, usually by giving single doses to healthy volunteers. Would the same results be found if the medications were given over a period of weeks or months? What if the person were older and had other health problems? What if he or she were taking seven other

(Continued)

(*Continued*)

medications? Most of these questions remain inadequately answered. There are also valid reasons for thinking AEDs are special, compared with many other drugs. Some AEDs have a narrow range between a toxic dose (too high) and an ineffective dose (too low). Thus even small changes in blood levels might be meaningful. Also, the nature of epilepsy is different from other medical conditions. If a change in a blood pressure medication to generic results in the blood pressure being a few points higher, there may be no immediate consequences. However, if a change to a generic seizure medication results in a breakthrough seizure, the consequences can be dire for work, driving, and safety.

What information do we have that is specific to generic AEDs? Several lines of evidence suggest that AEDs are different than other classes of medications. First, numerous reports from patients and providers have documented breakthrough seizures resulting from changes to generic AEDs. However, epilepsy is a variable condition, and people might be more prone to report seizures close to the time of a medication change and ignore others.

In some countries, such as Canada, switches to generic medications were required. If unsuccessful, a return to the brand name medication could be requested (a "switchback"). Researchers found that the switchback rates for AEDs were much higher than for other drugs, such as antidepressants or heart medicines. These studies also supported that AEDs were special, although fears and biases on the part of patients or providers still could have been causing the higher switchback rates.

A few studies have looked at what actually happened to groups of people whose AEDs were changed. One study from

(*Continued*)

(*Continued*)

Canada compared those who stayed on brand name medications to those who were switched among several different generic AEDs (some generics have 10 or more manufacturers). Not surprisingly they found that the group on generics had lower drug costs. However, those savings were more than offset by higher hospital costs in those treated with generics. The generics-treated group had more fractures and more head injuries. Similar findings were seen in a US study.

Additional studies are needed before firm conclusions can be drawn. In the meantime, it remains an area of controversy. What conclusions, or at least considerations, can be drawn?

If you have new-onset seizures or are undergoing AED changes, generic medications may be a reasonable consideration. If you are taking an AED for which it is difficult to keep stable levels, such as phenytoin, generic substitution can be more problematic. For people like Jerry who have had good control of their seizures for a long time, switches to generic medications should be avoided if at all possible. If a change to a generic medication is made, seizure control should be tracked carefully. It is often helpful to have baseline AED levels checked before and after the change, adjusting dose if needed. Whenever possible, frequent changes between generics produced by different manufacturers should be avoided.

Chapter 10

Side Effects

In all antiepileptic drug (AED) decisions, the issue of potential side effects (sometimes called adverse effects) should be part of the discussion. Often, when several choices of treatment are available, your doctor may consider possible side effects to be the biggest factor in AED choice, especially when differences in effectiveness are small. This chapter will address the most common side effects associated with both the short- and long-term use of AEDs, as well as some rarer but potentially serious ones. Sometimes problems arise from interactions between different medications, so common drug-drug interactions and the need for medication monitoring will be discussed.

You can probably imagine that a discussion of medication side effects could be quite detailed. Anyone who has heard a medication advertisement on television knows that half of the advertisement seems to be a list of possible side effects! If you research a medication on the Internet or look at the detailed information that comes in the package, you could easily be overwhelmed by the amount of information listed *for just a single drug*. What is often missing is any sense of proportion. How common is dizziness? What are the chances that a liver problem could occur? How many people have tingling of their left fourth toe? Okay, the last one is a little silly, but some of these lists of side effects are quite detailed. There is usually a general requirement that *any* side effect that occurs during study of a medication be reported, regardless of whether it was directly produced by the medication.

How can we best process all of this information? In this section, I'd like to give you a basic framework for thinking about AED side effects. I'll break them up into three categories:

- Acute (usually related to the amount of drug taken and reversible if the dose is reduced)
- Idiosyncratic (less common, less predictable, and sometimes serious)
- Chronic (sometimes appearing after many years of use; seriousness and reversibility may vary)

I will focus on *categories* of side effects. Along the way, I will mention some specific drugs that may be more likely to produce that side effect, but I will try to steer clear of listing each drug and all of its potential side effects. You can use Appendix 2 to look up specific drugs, and some common side effects (not an exhaustive list) are included there.

Acute (Usually Dose-Related and Reversible) Side Effects of AEDs

AEDs are designed to work on the brain. The goal is to block the abnormal, rapid firing of brain cells that occurs during a seizure while leaving normal brain function unaffected. This approach is common in medical therapy—antibiotics try to kill the infection while leaving human cells unaffected. Cancer chemotherapy tries to target the rapidly dividing cancer cells while leaving normal cell division unaffected. In each of these examples, the treatment is not completely selective for disease. In other words, sometimes normal function, not just the disease condition, can be affected by drugs.

Since AEDs work on the brain, it is not surprising, then, that the most common side effects are neurologic or psychiatric. The drugs target seizures, but especially at high doses they may "spill over" and affect some normal brain functions. What side effects should you watch for?

Common brain-related side effects of AEDs include sleepiness or fatigue, unsteadiness or dizziness, tremor (shakiness), or tingling. Some AEDs at high doses, especially the related drugs carbamazepine (Tegretol), oxcarbazepine (Trileptal), and eslicarbazepine (Aptiom), can cause blurry or double vision. This often occurs when the medication level is at a peak after a dose is absorbed. It generally goes away if the dose is reduced or if a longer-acting, extended-release preparation of carbamazepine or oxcarbazepine is used to eliminate some of the peak dose effects. Eslicarbazepine is inherently a long-acting drug and does not require an extended release form. A general feeling of mental slowing is possible with several of the AEDs, especially at high doses. In most cases, overall intelligence does not change, but processing speed and mental quickness are more commonly affected. Some of my patients report a mild version of this. They may not see it as a problem but, if asked, might note that "things just don't click" as quickly or that they feel a "half-step slower." At other times, this side effect is clearly in the range of causing problems. Reducing the dose can sometimes eliminate this side effect. If it does not, a change to a different AED may be needed. This was exactly what Derek experienced.

Derek worked in the business world and frequently had to do presentations and public speaking that required him to "think on his feet." When he developed epilepsy, his seizures were quickly controlled with medication, but he felt like the medication was affecting his work performance. He felt less confident and less quick to respond when presenting his ideas at work. In this situation, Derek made a good choice. He did not reduce or stop his medication on his own, which would

(Continued)

(Continued)
have put him at risk for more seizures. Instead, he discussed the issue with his neurologist. After considering a number of factors besides medication that might have been contributing (such as stress and poor sleep), Derek's doctor concluded that he probably was having problems as a result of his AED. They planned a gradual switch to an alternative medication, and Derek also started to take a little extra time to prepare for his presentations at work. As a result of these two changes, Derek felt like he was at the top of his game again.

The brain is not all about thinking but also about feeling and mood. Problems with mood are very common in people with epilepsy, as is discussed in Chapter 3. Often this is a result of the biology of having epilepsy: Brain regions responsible for mood are affected by seizures. Social limitations as a result of epilepsy may play a smaller role. In some cases, AED therapy can also cause or worsen mood problems. It is difficult to make a reliable list of those AEDs most prone to causing mood difficulties as the responses are somewhat individual. Among the older AEDs, the barbiturates (phenobarbital, primidone) are known for this potential effect, and this is one reason their use has been reduced in recent times. Among the newer drugs, mood problems can also be seen. Sometimes this takes the form of depression and at other times irritability. These issues are seen somewhat more commonly with certain medications, including topiramate (Topamax), levetiracetam (Keppra), zonisamide (Zonegran), and perampanel (Fycompa). Some less commonly prescribed AEDs may also be more likely to show these mood effects, including tiagabine (Gabitril), vigabatrin (Sabril), and felbamate (Felbatol). Mood problems are *not* unique to these drugs and can potentially be seen with any AED. When starting or changing the dose of an AED, it is important to be alert to any mood changes, including new or worsening suicidal thoughts.

Debates in Epilepsy: AEDs and Suicidality

As a group, all of the AEDs carry a US Food and Drug Administration (FDA) warning for possible increase in suicidality. That is alarming to many people, especially because in most cases *not* using an AED is not a viable option. Since the FDA warning appeared in 2008, many epilepsy experts have had mixed feelings and have expressed concerns.

On the one hand, there is recognition that this is a serious issue. Suicidal thoughts and actions *are* more common in people with epilepsy than in the general public, for reasons explored in Chapter 3. This issue deserves attention. Yet many epilepsy experts have also expressed concerns about the way that warnings were applied across the board to all AEDs.

How did the FDA come to this conclusion? They looked at 199 studies of 11 different AEDs, in which some participants received an AED and others received placebo (an inactive compound, like a sugar pill). Only about one-quarter of people in these studies had epilepsy; many others were receiving AEDs in studies of pain, migraine, or psychiatric disease. They looked at how many people *reported* suicidal thoughts or actions in the course of the study. These symptoms were reported in small numbers of participants—less than 1 percent of both groups—but were about twice as common in people receiving AEDs than those receiving placebo. That sounds like a lot! But it needs to be put into perspective.

Because these reports were so rare in both groups, it was calculated that one additional case of suicidal thinking or behavior would be expected for every 530 people treated with an AED. When stated this way, it still sounds concerning but less alarming.

(Continued)

(*Continued*)

Other questions were raised. People were not actively asked about suicidal thoughts or behaviors in these studies—they had to volunteer them. There was concern that those receiving AEDs might have had more contact with the researchers (because they might have been more prone overall to other sorts of side effects if taking an active drug) and therefore would have had more opportunities to report suicidal thoughts. This could make the numbers look artificially high in the AED group. Second, the report lumps all AEDs together, when in fact good evidence exists that some may have positive mood effects and others negative effects.

Mood problems are common in epilepsy, and suicidality is a very serious issue. When starting a new AED, it is important to watch for any mood changes. But the small possible risk of worsening mood also needs to be kept in perspective. It is much more dangerous to stop seizure medication out of fear of side effects. If you or your family notice mood changes, you should talk with your doctor right away. There are often many options for changing your AED if needed. It may also be helpful to seek help from a mental health professional, at least for a period of time.

Before we leave the topic of brain-related side effects, it is worth mentioning that changes in sexual interest or function can be related to AEDs. As with mood problems, sexual dysfunction can sometimes be a part of the underlying epilepsy and seizures rather than the AEDs used to treat it. However, there is little doubt that some AEDs can add to the problem. Problems have been most commonly reported with use of the older AEDs. Specifically, problems are most often seen with medications called **enzyme-inducing AEDs**, or **EIAEDs**. This is likely because these drugs can cause more rapid breakdown of sex hormones, such as testosterone. They may also contribute to sexual problems by other means.

With regard to changes in sexual interest or function, there are a few important things to remember. First, sexual dysfunction in people with epilepsy is fairly common and can have several causes— AEDs are just one of these. If you are having concerns about sexual dysfunction, *tell your doctor*. Although not always the case, some studies have shown that providers are reluctant to bring up issues of sexual health, so it is important for you to advocate for yourself. Your doctor, or in some cases a specialist that you may be referred to, should look broadly for possible causes. If this evaluation suggests that AEDs are playing an important role, reduction in dose or change to another AED should be considered.

Although AEDs work on the brain, they can also produce side effects in other body systems. Here are some of the more common areas:

Gastrointestinal: GI problems are not very common. Some AEDs can cause nausea, heartburn, or diarrhea/loose stools, including valproic acid (Depakene).

Weight gain or loss: Many AEDs are weight neutral—they don't commonly cause weight changes—but some can. For some people weight loss might be seen as a positive side effect, although for others it can be a major problem and a reason to stop the medication. AEDs that commonly produce some weight gain include sodium valproate or valproic acid (Depakote or Depakene), pregabalin (Lyrica), and, to a lesser extent, gabapentin (Neurontin) and carbamazepine (Tegretol). AEDs that commonly produce some weight *loss* include topiramate (Topamax), zonisamide (Zonegran), and felbamate (Felbatol).

Changes detected on blood tests: When you are taking AEDs, your doctor may periodically check blood tests. Sometimes mild abnormalities are seen on these tests that do not require any intervention other than periodic monitoring. Rarely, blood tests may identify a serious problem requiring change of AED dose or of the AED altogether.

Decreases in the level of sodium in the bloodstream can be seen with the use of carbamazepine (Tegretol) and its relatives, oxcarbazepine (Trileptal) and eslicarbazepine (Aptiom). These changes can be seen in anyone taking these medications, but they are more frequent and sometimes more severe in older people. Mild decreases in the sodium level are common with the use of these drugs and usually do not require anything more than periodic monitoring. More substantial decreases in blood sodium may require limiting water intake, reducing the dose of the offending medication, or even changing to a different AED. Severe decreases in blood sodium can be dangerous and can cause neurologic problems, including more seizures. Careful action, often involving hospitalization and slow, careful correction of the sodium level, needs to be taken in these severe cases.

Many AEDs are processed in the liver, and blood tests are done to assess for the rare possibility of liver problems. Commonly, some of these liver tests may be slightly elevated in people taking AEDs. Mild elevations are not unexpected and often do not require any action. When elevated by more than two to three times the upper range of normal for the lab, it could signal a more serious issue and, depending on the circumstance, may trigger more frequent lab monitoring, a change in AED dose, or a change in the AED used for treatment.

Decreases in blood counts are sometimes seen with AED use. A low white blood cell count can be seen with use of several AEDs, including carbamazepine (Tegretol). This is often mild and may not require any action; rarely it is more marked and triggers a change in therapy. Severe problems with blood counts have been seen with felbamate (Felbatol), and this will be discussed more in the next section. Decreases in platelets are seen fairly commonly in people taking sodium valproate or valproic acid (Depakote or Depakene). Platelets are a component of the blood that promotes blood clotting. If the platelet count is low, it could result in easy bruising or bleeding—for example, nosebleeds or bleeding gums. Low platelets with sodium valproate/valproic acid use is usually dose related. It is often seen at higher doses and often gets better with decreases in the dose. If the decrease in platelet count is mild and not causing any symptoms, as is often the case, nothing may need to be done. More marked decreases, especially if associated with bleeding problems, usually require dose reductions or medication change.

Idiosyncratic Side Effects

The word idiosyncratic is often defined as something that is characteristic of a single person. It is something that is unique, or relatively unique, to that person. With medications, it often refers to an unusual individual reaction to a drug.

Therefore, idiosyncratic side effects are relatively rare, unexpected side effects seen in a relatively small number of individuals. Although rare, they can sometimes be quite serious. It is important to be aware of some of these possible reactions so that you can report them to your doctor or get emergency care right away.

The most common idiosyncratic side effects with AEDs are allergic reactions to drugs. Usually these appear after the first several weeks or months of use, but they can appear later, especially following dose changes. The reaction is caused by the body seeing the drug as something foreign and potentially dangerous, triggering an immune reaction. In the course of this reaction, the body is affected by the immune response as an "innocent bystander" in the battle between the immune system and the drug. Most frequently, allergic reactions take the form of a rash, although the liver and other organ systems can be involved. If not identified and treated promptly, these reactions can be very serious and even life threatening. The names of some of these feared reactions include **Stevens-Johnson syndrome (SJS)** and **toxic epidermal necrolysis (TEN)**. Symptoms often begin nonspecifically, with fever, fatigue, or sore throat. The process then progresses to produce ulcers of the mouth and eyes and a widespread rash across the body with loss of a layer of skin much like with a burn injury. Some tests are now becoming available to help identify those who may be genetically prone to these reactions (see Chapter 7). Many AEDs can potentially provoke these reactions, including, but not limited to, phenobarbital, phenytoin, carbamazepine, lamotrigine (especially in children), oxcarbazepine, and clobazam. Until testing becomes more advanced, the best defense is education. If you are started on one of these medications and have this reaction, you should contact your doctor immediately. Your doctor may need to get you off of the medication quickly and treat the allergic reaction to avoid serious problems.

Mild decreases in blood counts was mentioned in the last section as a possible and usually manageable side effect of therapy with some AEDs. Rarely, a more serious idiosyncratic reaction can be seen. Most of the blood cells are produced inside the large bones, in the bone marrow. Rarely, certain drugs can cause the bone marrow to shut down. This can cause many problems, including infection (from too few white blood cells), fatigue and anemia (from too few red blood cells), and bleeding (from too few platelets). This is a very rare reaction to AED therapy. After the introduction of felbamate (Felbatol) in the 1990s, several cases of this reaction, called "aplastic anemia," were seen, including severe forms causing death. The risk of aplastic anemia in patients taking felbamate is estimated to be 100 times greater than in the general population. Felbamate was not taken off of the market, but its use is very limited to situations where the benefit is felt to outweigh the risk. To use felbamate, a consent process is required to ensure that someone being started understands the risks. This is one of the important reasons that your doctor may do blood tests to monitor your blood counts. It is important to follow through with all required testing so that any of these rare reactions can be detected and treated early.

Serious liver problems can result from an idiosyncratic reaction to AEDs. This is very rare. This problem has been seen following treatment with sodium valproate or valproic acid (Depakote or Depakene), especially in very young children. Felbamate (Felbatol) use has also been associated with a higher risk of liver failure. Serious liver problems resulting from use of other AEDs is exceedingly rare. If you have severe nausea, vomiting, or see a change in your skin color, you should tell your doctor right away, as these could be signs of a liver problem. A number of the newer AEDs largely avoid this issue by being primarily or exclusively cleared by the kidneys, with minimal or no processing by the liver. These include levetiracetam (Keppra), gabapentin (Neurontin), pregabalin (Lyrica), lacosamide (Vimpat), and eslicarbazepine (Aptiom). If you have known liver disease, your doctor may preferentially choose one of these medications for you.

Chronic Side Effects

Chronic side effects are those that may appear after many years of use. The seriousness and reversibility of these side effects may vary.

Long-term use of phenytoin (Dilantin) can cause slowly progressive loss of sensation in the feet in some people (neuropathy). After years of phenytoin use, brain scans may show that a portion of the back of the brain called the cerebellum is smaller as a result of chronic drug exposure. Chronic phenytoin use can also cause excessive hair growth, coarsening of facial features, and overgrowth of the gums.

Use of the AED vigabatrin (Sabril) has been limited by the potential risk to vision. A gradual loss of peripheral vision can be seen as an effect of dosing this drug for months or years. Because of this, vigabatrin is only available through a special program that includes education and regular visual testing.

Multiple other possible chronic side effects on other body systems are discussed elsewhere in this book, including effects on bone health (osteoporosis) and the possibility of producing birth defects in pregnant women.

Given the large number of AEDs, it is not practical or wise to try to list every possible side effect of every AED. You should discuss any concerns about long-term or other side effects of your AEDs with your doctor.

Medication Interactions

You are probably already aware that taking several different medications together can sometimes be problematic. Interactions between medications can sometimes boost the level of one of the medications (risk for toxicity) or reduce the levels of the affected medication (risk for ineffective treatment). AEDs are no exception to this problem. In fact, some of the older (and a few of the newer) AEDs are among the most troublesome for medication interactions.

Many drug interactions happen as part of the metabolism, or breakdown, of medications in the body. Some medications are called **inducers**. These medications act on the liver to *speed up* the breakdown of some other medications. The opposite effect can also happen—medications that are **inhibitors** act on the liver to *slow down* the breakdown of other medications. These inducers or inhibitors can influence the breakdown of a large number of other compounds. The older AEDs tend to have effects on many other drugs. Some newer AEDs are inducers or inhibitors, but they tend to affect a more limited number of other drugs.

If you look at a list of drugs that are inducers and inhibitors, you will see a lot of AEDs listed! This means that these medications have a high potential to interact with other drugs—both AEDs and non-AEDs. This does not mean that they can't be used. It is usually possible to account for the interaction and adjust dosing, but it does make things more complicated problems more prone to occur (Box 10–1).

BOX 10-1 AEDs That Influence the Breakdown
of Other Medications

*Some AEDs That Speed Up the Breakdown
of Other Medications (Inducers)*

Phenobarbital
Primidone
Phenytoin
Carbamazepine
Oxcarbazepine
Eslicarbazepine
Topiramate
Felbamate

*Some AEDs That Slow the Breakdown of Other
Medications (Inhibitors)*

Sodium Valproate/Valproic Acid
Felbamate
Topiramate
Oxcarbazepine

Medication interactions can happen in several different scenarios. Most people recognize that medication interactions can occur when a drug that is an inhibitor or inducer is added to an existing mix of medications. This is indeed a common situation, and the doses of the other drugs may need to be adjusted. But there are other situations to consider.

If an inducer is *already* on the medication list—for example, imagine that someone is already taking phenytoin—then any other medication that is acted on by phenytoin will be affected in that person. If a cholesterol-lowering medication is added, it will be broken down more quickly because of the presence of phenytoin, and the dose may need to be doubled just to get a normal effect.

The least considered situation is when an inhibitor or inducer is stopped. For example, let's consider someone who is taking phenytoin and a blood thinner. Phenytoin induces (speeds up) the breakdown of the blood thinner, but the dose of the blood thinner has been adjusted (increased) to account for this. Now the neurologist decides to discontinue phenytoin in favor of another AED that is not an inducer. When the phenytoin is taken away, the effects of the blood thinner will be much greater and might cause bleeding problems if not adjusted downward.

The list of drugs that can be induced or inhibited by AEDs is long. This includes AEDs themselves but also other very important medications such as birth control pills, HIV medications, cancer chemotherapy, blood thinners, and vitamins. Again, these interactions can often be anticipated and accounted for. Electronic databases help doctors, nurses, and pharmacists spot potential problems. But life would be simpler if we just didn't have to worry about them. So in general, it is favorable if an AED is neither an inducer nor an inhibitor.

Some AEDs are not processed by the liver at all (or are minimally processed) and get around much of the issue of medication interactions. This makes them easier to use if you are taking other medications. These AEDs include gabapentin, pregabalin, levetiracetam, lacosamide, and eslicarbazepine.

Monitoring

With nearly every AED on the market, it is possible to check a blood level. The blood level tells your doctor how much of the medication is in the bloodstream. People of different sizes and rates of metabolism may require different AED doses. But what is most important is not the dose, but the end result—the amount of medication in the bloodstream. Simplistically, this can be thought of as:

(Amount of drug given) − (amount of drug metabolized or cleared) = blood level.

Although monitoring the levels of AEDs is important, your doctor may not need to check them frequently. Most AED dosing decisions are made on a clinical basis—based on how the person is doing—rather than on a number obtained from a blood test. There is a saying that doctors use: "Treat the patient, not the number." If you have no side effects but have continued seizures, your doctor will likely want to increase your AED regardless of the blood level number. If you are having side effects, your doctor will likely reduce your dose or change the AED regardless of the number shown on a blood test.

Having said that, there are several specific situations in which your doctor may want to check your AED levels.

- Establishing a benchmark—a level at which your seizures are well controlled. This can be a useful reference point for comparison should a breakthrough seizure occur.
- Optimizing AED therapy. Sometimes knowing the level can help to fine-tune dosing.
- Assessing whether the medication is being taken as directed. If your AED level is zero, it may prompt your doctor to sit down with you and explore whether there are barriers to taking your medication regularly.
- Teasing out drug–drug interactions. If you are taking multiple medications that might interact, levels can be a useful guidepost.
- Monitoring during pregnancy. As we will see in Chapter 13, blood levels of AEDs can sometimes change dramatically with

all of the physical changes of pregnancy, and close monitoring of levels during pregnancy is often helpful.

In addition to checking AED levels, periodic screening tests of blood chemistries, blood counts, and liver and kidney function are often performed. In general, your doctor might check these to establish a baseline before starting a new AED, again a few weeks to months after starting a new AED, and then often annually thereafter. Your doctor might check these screening tests sooner if symptoms occur that suggest problems with one of these systems. This last practice—checking your screening blood tests annually—is of uncertain benefit in detecting AED-related problems but is still often common practice.

Chapter 11

Beyond AEDs

Surgical Therapy

We have seen that approximately two-thirds of people with epilepsy are able to obtain adequate control of seizures using antiepileptic drugs (AEDs) without substantial side effects. In the remaining one-third of people with epilepsy, however, seizures persist despite all efforts with medical therapy. If you are in this situation or know someone who is, you will want to learn more about the other options for treatment discussed in this chapter. If you have focal-onset seizures, you might be a candidate for epilepsy surgery. Evaluation for epilepsy surgery involves precisely identifying the seizure focus and determining if removal of that focus would be a safe and effective means of treating the epilepsy.

> Twenty-eight-year-old Robert had been experiencing difficulty controlling his seizures since age 25. His initial diagnosis of epilepsy actually came much earlier. He had a seizure associated with high fever (**febrile seizure**) as a child that was prolonged, lasting nearly 45 minutes, and requiring hospitalization. He had no further seizures until age 13, when he began experiencing complex partial seizures. After having several seizures, his epilepsy came under control on carbamazepine (Tegretol) and was something that he didn't think about often. He just visited his neurologist for an annual checkup and to renew his prescription.
>
> (*Continued*)

(Continued)

At age 25, for unclear reasons, something changed for Robert. He was at work and felt the odd feeling in the pit of his stomach that used to accompany his seizures. The next thing he knew, his boss and coworkers were around him and paramedics were preparing to take him to the hospital. He was told that he had been staring and unresponsive, but he had no memory of the event at all. When the same thing happened at home a few days later, his doctor increased his carbamazepine dose. Unfortunately, the seizures continued. His neurologist changed his medication to lamotrigine (Lamictal). He was able to tolerate high doses of this medication better than the carbamazepine, but he continued having complex partial seizures once or twice per month on average; some months he had three to four seizures. Levetiracetam (Keppra) was added to the lamotrigine, with slight benefit, but seizures still continued. His neurologist repeated a brain MRI scan since the last one performed had been in his teenage years. The MRI showed atrophy (smaller size) in the middle portion of the right temporal lobe called the **hippocampus**. The finding was suggestive of **mesial temporal sclerosis**, an abnormality of the hippocampus that can result from a number of childhood injuries, such as infection, head trauma, or prolonged febrile seizures like the kind Robert had experienced. Robert's routine EEG showed sharp waves in the right temporal lobe.

Now, at age 28, he was missing work frequently because of seizures. He was not able to drive. He asked his neurologist if there was another medication that could do a better job of controlling his seizures. The answer surprised him. His neurologist told him that the chances of getting complete seizure control with further medication trials was small. He recommended that Robert undergo more testing to see if he might

(Continued)

> (*Continued*)
>
> be a candidate for epilepsy surgery. With the right findings on these tests, he might have a very high chance of being seizure free following epilepsy surgery. This was the part that really surprised Robert because he had always thought that epilepsy surgery was a "last resort" treatment when everything else had failed.

Robert's neurologist was right—he was potentially an excellent candidate for epilepsy surgery. Let's spend a few moments thinking about what people are considered candidates for epilepsy surgery.

Epilepsy Surgery

Candidates for Epilepsy Surgery

The first step is usually to determine whether a person has **medically refractory** or medication-resistant epilepsy. This simply means deciding whether or not seizures can be controlled with AED therapy. If seizures *can* be controlled with AEDs, a person is not usually considered to be a candidate for epilepsy surgery, barring the exceptional circumstances described hereafter.

Deciding whether someone has medically refractory epilepsy is not quite as simple as it sounds. Making this determination after someone has had uncontrolled seizures for 20 years and after 12 different AED trials is not so difficult. But that is not the goal. The goal is *early* identification of medically refractory epilepsy, so that futile additional trials of AEDs are not pursued and so that other forms of more effective therapy may be explored early, rather than after 20 years of uncontrolled epilepsy.

Several studies now suggest that medically refractory epilepsy can be identified early. In people who have continued seizures despite trials of two or three appropriate AEDs, the chances of gaining complete control of seizures with additional AED trials is generally small, probably less than 10 percent in most cases. People who continue to have seizures after trying two or more AEDs should talk to their doctors about other approaches, including evaluation for epilepsy surgery. If the initial AED trials were limited by side effects (in other words, if effective doses could not be reached because of side effects), the chances that a person will become seizure free with more AED trials is somewhat more hopeful. But if those first two to three drugs were correctly chosen and were used at typically effective doses but were unsuccessful in controlling your seizures, the outlook for complete seizure control with additional trials is not good. When an individual has longstanding, poorly controlled focal seizures, the outlook is even poorer. Studies of new AEDs often enroll people with long-term, poorly controlled seizures. In these studies, the number of people who become seizure free with the new AED added is very small, less than 5 percent (less than 1 in 20 people) in nearly every study. Thus there seems to be something different about medically refractory epilepsy that can often be identified early so that other treatment considerations, including epilepsy surgery, can be explored.

There are occasional exceptions to the rule of surgical candidates having medically refractory epilepsy. When a person is seizure free but seizure control was achieved only on high doses of multiple medications with prominent side effects, surgery might still be considered if testing shows a high likelihood of seizure freedom. When a brain tumor or abnormal blood vessel in the brain that might bleed is a cause of seizures, surgery might be considered even though the seizures are controlled with medication. In such a setting, control of seizures with the surgery may be an important, but secondary, issue.

Is everyone with medically refractory epilepsy a possible surgical candidate? The answer to this is no. In most instances, epilepsy surgery is only considered if a person has focal epilepsy—simple partial, complex partial, or secondarily generalized seizures. In these syndromes, there is the possibility of locating a seizure focus and making a determination of whether the focus is safe to surgically remove to treat the epilepsy. The process of making this determination is discussed next.

People with genetic, generalized epilepsy are not candidates for epilepsy surgery. With these syndromes, there is no seizure focus to remove. Instead, the gene changes produce an overall tendency throughout the brain to have seizures. Fortunately this group of epilepsies is more responsive to treatment with AEDs and less often medically refractory. Much less commonly, a different type of epilepsy surgery is considered in people with symptomatic generalized epilepsies such as Lennox-Gastaut syndrome (LGS), as discussed in the next section.

Common Surgically Treatable Epilepsies

Certainly not everyone with medically refractory focal epilepsy will turn out to be a good surgical candidate. However, experience has shown that certain patterns of epilepsy have somewhat predictable responses to surgery. Keep in mind that these approximate numbers apply to large groups of people who have undergone the described surgery. You will want to discuss the unique features of your epilepsy with your doctor.

Mesial Temporal Sclerosis

This syndrome, mentioned previously, involves injury and scarring to the middle part of the temporal lobe, affecting a structure called the hippocampus and sometimes other neighboring structures. Sometimes the cause of MTS is known (for example, an old injury from childhood meningitis or a prolonged febrile seizure). Often the cause is not known with certainty. Seizures may include simple partial seizures (auras), complex partial seizures, and secondarily generalized tonic-clonic seizures. Typical findings on MRI include atrophy (loss of tissue) in the medial temporal lobe and often increased (bright) signal, indicating scarring. Interictal EEG shows abnormal discharges (spikes or sharp waves) in the temporal lobe, and video-EEG monitoring shows seizures of temporal lobe onset.

This syndrome usually responds poorly to AED therapy. When the typical pattern is seen and the findings from testing all match and point to the same focus, the chances of seizure freedom after surgery can be very high: the best outcome of any epilepsy surgery. Most studies report an approximately 80 percent chance of being seizure free in the first years following surgery for MTS. Some people may have rare seizures many years after surgery or with attempted discontinuation of medication, bringing the long-term seizure-free rate closer to 65 percent.

Other Temporal Lobe Epilepsy

Epilepsy surgery is also frequently performed in people who have medically refractory temporal lobe epilepsy but *not* MTS. The majority of these people have seizures that begin in the mesial temporal region. However, some others may have seizure onset in other parts of the temporal lobe. In some cases, a cause for the seizures, such as a developmental abnormality of the temporal lobe, a low-grade tumor, or a blood vessel malformation, can be clearly seen on MRI. Sometimes no abnormality can be seen on MRI even though other tests strongly suggest that the temporal lobe is the focus. If all testing identifies the same temporal lobe focus, people with medically refractory temporal lobe epilepsy not caused by MTS also do very well with epilepsy surgery. Approximately 50 to 70 percent will be seizure free following surgery.

Extratemporal Epilepsy

Most epilepsy surgery is done in people with temporal lobe epilepsy. However, seizures may also start in other parts of the brain (Figure 11–1), and many of these people may also be candidates for

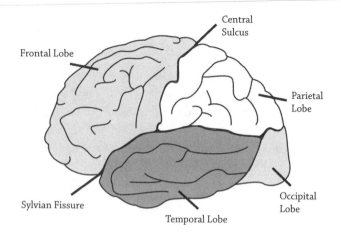

FIGURE 11-1 Major divisions of the brain into lobes. Reproduced with permission from Caplan, L. *Navigating the Complexities of Stroke.* © American Academy of Neurology 2013.

surgery if the seizures do not respond to AEDs. **Extratemporal epilepsy** is the term for seizures that start outside the temporal lobe. The second most common site for seizure onset is the frontal lobe. Less often, seizures may begin in the parietal or occipital lobes.

Localizing seizures that begin outside of the temporal lobes can sometimes be more difficult. When a person has difficult-to-control seizures that start outside of the temporal lobe, the doctor and surgery team can order additional tests to determine whether surgical treatment of the epilepsy is an option. Sometimes more detailed, intracranial EEG recordings (testing with electrodes placed in or on the surface of the brain) are needed.

In general, when an extratemporal seizure focus is seen on MRI, all tests agree that this is the focus, and the abnormality can be safely removed, seizure-free outcomes can be high—in the range of 50 to 70 percent. When no abnormality is seen on MRI, or when other tests are less certain about the focus and intracranial monitoring is required, the outcomes are less favorable, often with less than 50 percent of people becoming seizure free after surgery.

Other Epilepsy Surgery

Much less commonly, epilepsy surgery is done without a goal of seizure freedom. In some limited instances, the goals are more modest, with the hope of simply reducing seizures or reducing the most disabling seizure types.

Corpus Callosotomy

This surgery is sometimes performed in children with Lennox-Gastaut syndrome (LGS) and severe seizures of multiple types, including drop seizures. Although the focus of this book is not childhood epilepsy, adolescents or adults with LGS are occasionally candidates for this procedure, as well. In these people, a single seizure focus cannot be identified. However, certain of the seizure types experienced are not truly generalized at onset, but result from rapid spread of the seizure discharge from one half of the brain to the other. This is especially the case for certain of the most disabling seizure types that people with LGS may experience: drop seizures (tonic and atonic seizures). Drop seizures often cause injuries from falls related to the sudden loss of muscle tone from an atonic seizure or the sudden stiffening and inability to maintain posture that happens with tonic seizures.

When these seizures cannot be controlled with AEDs, a different type of epilepsy surgery, with different goals, is sometimes considered. This surgery is called a **corpus callosotomy**. With this surgery, the goal is not to remove the seizure focus. Since this type of epilepsy has no single seizure focus, removing the focus is not possible. Instead, the surgery cuts a bundle of fibers ("wires") that connects the two halves, or hemispheres, of the brain called the **corpus callosum**. Often this surgery can block the rapid spread of seizure discharges from one half of the brain to the other and may markedly decrease seizures—especially the dangerous drop seizures. The goals are different here. There is little chance of seizure freedom with corpus callosotomy. Instead, the goal is to reduce the number of the most disabling seizure types and improve quality of life.

It might sound like this surgery would have dire consequences. In fact, there are some important risks to be aware of. Many children do remarkably well with recovery from corpus callosotomy; adolescents and adults are more likely to have long-lasting consequences. The most common, and often temporary, changes seen are a decrease in speech output and other language difficulties and symptoms that arise from disconnection of the two halves of the brain. This "disconnection syndrome" can be quite striking. For example, one hand may try to button up a shirt, while the other is trying to unbutton it. Fortunately these symptoms are often short-lived, and, amazingly, detailed testing may be required in people later on to demonstrate any effects of the surgery.

Corpus callosotomy can sometimes produce a dramatic decrease in drop seizures, but seizures of other types typically persist. This approach is very different from removal of a seizure focus, on which most of the subsequent discussion will focus.

Is Epilepsy Surgery Effective?

For many years, studies described groups of patients who benefited from epilepsy surgery. Series of patients who had undergone surgery and became seizure free were reported. While this evidence seemed convincing, reports of this type are more prone to error, including a placebo response. The placebo response is seen when an ineffective treatment appears to improve the medical condition, in part because of the expectations of the patient, family, and medical team. You might think there is little chance of placebo response in something like epilepsy, where seizures can be counted. However, you would be wrong. Most studies of new AEDs show a clear placebo response, often accounting for 20 to 30 percent of the seizure reduction from treatment. When a major treatment such as surgery is done, the chance of finding a placebo response is especially high. In medical science, the strongest proof that a treatment is effective comes from a **randomized controlled trial (RCT)**. In these studies, participants are randomly assigned (as by a coin toss) to either active treatment (the medication or surgery being studied) or to a placebo (a sugar pill, or no surgery), and results from the two groups are compared. If those in the active treatment group do better than those in the placebo group, the evidence is scientifically convincing for the new treatment.

In some situations it is very difficult to do a randomized controlled trial. You might imagine that epilepsy surgery is one of those conditions. How could you take a group of people who are candidates for epilepsy surgery and tell half of them that they would not have surgery because they are in the "placebo" group? That would be unethical. This is the main reason that for many years this most convincing form of evidence for epilepsy surgery was lacking.

This changed when some researchers used a feature of the Canadian health care system to their advantage to study epilepsy surgery in people with temporal lobe epilepsy—the most common type of epilepsy surgery. At that time, there was a waiting list for people who were found to be candidates for temporal lobe epilepsy surgery. To conduct the study, half of these people were randomly assigned to immediate surgical treatment. The others continued on best AED therapy for one year until their names came up for surgery on the usual wait list. The researchers compared the immediate surgery group to the "best medical therapy" group (those who were still waiting for surgery). The results were very convincing.

Of the group who underwent surgery, nearly two-thirds (64 percent) became seizure free, compared with 8 percent of those treated with best AED therapy. That is a big difference! The surgery proved to be quite safe. Not only were the seizures more effectively stopped, but quality-of-life measures also favored the immediate surgery group. Other studies have confirmed this finding and suggested that early surgery is better than waiting and trying medications for many years.

With these convincing findings, you might assume that everyone eligible for epilepsy surgery is being evaluated and treated.

In fact, there is great concern among epilepsy experts that epilepsy surgery is an underutilized treatment. Why would this be? For many years, undertreatment was attributed to lack of randomized controlled studies and lack of guidelines for neurologists from national associations. However, the first randomized controlled trials of epilepsy surgery were published more than 10 years ago. Following this, in 2003, the American Academy of Neurology (supported by the American Epilepsy Society and the American Association of Neurological Surgeons) published clearly worded "practice parameters," or guidelines, for use of epilepsy surgery. These guidelines stated that patients with temporal lobe epilepsy should be "referred to a surgical epilepsy center on failing appropriate first-line antiepileptic drugs." Discouragingly, a recent study looked at referral patterns for epilepsy surgery in the years before the guidelines, and then again 10 years after the publication of the guidelines. Little had changed. It appeared that epilepsy surgery was still underutilized, and, on average, AED therapy was tried for 17 to 18 years before surgery was performed.

What other reasons could explain the slow and incomplete adoption of a highly effective therapy? There may be several. As we have seen, many new AEDs have become available in recent years, and some doctors (or patients) may feel inclined to pursue an ultimately futile effort to keep trying different AEDs for extended periods of time. Despite the evidence and guidelines, some doctors and many patients may not be aware of the effectiveness and safety of modern epilepsy surgery. In the United States, many people still have no or limited access to health care, which may also pose barriers to accessing appropriate care. Finally, it appears that there may be excessive fear of the risk of epilepsy surgery on the part of both patients and less experienced health care providers. The idea of brain surgery can be scary, and continuing to try different AEDs may seem "safer." In fact, the risk of epilepsy surgery must be weighed against the risk of continued refractory seizures, which is not small. As we will see, these risks can include high rates of injury, disability, poor quality of life, and measurably higher risk of sudden death.

Education of both patients and health care providers is needed. This education could put the benefits and risks of epilepsy surgery into context and may provide the best opportunity to change old patterns.

Who Should Be Considered for Epilepsy Surgery?

We have seen that epilepsy surgery can be highly effective, even when extensive trials of AEDs have failed. The ideal candidate for epilepsy surgery has medically refractory epilepsy that can be localized to a single focus that can be safely removed. The sought-after outcome is seizure freedom without introducing new problems as a result of the surgery.

Not everyone is an ideal candidate for surgery. For example, when more than one seizure focus exists, surgery generally cannot be safely done. In others, the focus may be located in an area of critical brain function that cannot be safely removed. And despite technological advances, sometimes the seizure focus still simply can't be securely located.

However, the evaluation process frequently leads to a safe and effective surgery that can result in seizure freedom despite years and sometimes decades of seizures that were not controlled with medications.

What is the process for identifying people who are most likely to benefit from epilepsy surgery? Much of the surgery evaluation process must be tailored to meet the needs of each individual. However, the next section discusses some common themes.

Standard Epilepsy Surgery Evaluation

This section describes the components of the evaluation that many, if not most, people with medically refractory epilepsy should undergo to help determine whether they are a potential candidate for epilepsy surgery:

- Careful neurologic history and examination
- MRI brain
- Video-EEG monitoring
- Neuropsychological testing

History and Examination

Just like the diagnosis of epilepsy, the evaluation for epilepsy surgery begins with a careful history and physical examination. Although it uses simple tools (for example, questions and a reflex hammer), it provides the core of the epilepsy surgery evaluation. When taking a history, the neurologist asks many questions, such as:

- When did the seizures start?
- How have they changed over time?
- What has been the response to trials of AEDs?
- Do you have any of the identified seizure risk factors, such as traumatic brain injury, stroke, or a family member with seizures?

The neurologist will want to know all about other medical conditions that have been diagnosed and all other medications that are taken. The neurologist will want to know how seizures have affected quality of life. Before considering surgery, the diagnosis of medically refractory epilepsy must be established. A careful review of the seizure history may provide strong clues to the area of seizure onset, which can guide further testing. The neurologic examination may identify findings that point to the area of the brain where seizures originate. Epilepsy surgery is definitely an area where technology does not provide all of the answers, and clues from a careful seizure history can be critically important.

Video-EEG and MRI

In addition to the questions and examination, two other studies will need to be done: MRI imaging of the brain and video-EEG monitoring. Both of these tests were discussed in Chapter 7. If the neurologist can identify a structural abnormality in the brain on MRI that might be responsible for the seizures, this abnormality can provide a target for the epilepsy surgeon and increase the likelihood that surgery will be successful in controlling seizures. Video-EEG monitoring helps identify where the electrical activity of a seizure begins. It is usually necessary to record several typical seizures to ensure that the same pattern of onset is seen with each seizure. If more than one seizure type is seen, additional recording may be needed to ensure that all seizure types are recorded.

Neuropsychological Testing

Neuropsychological testing is part of the standard evaluation for epilepsy surgery. The neuropsychologist will assess thinking, or cognitive function, during several hours of testing. The neuropsychologist will also ask about mood and psychological issues. This information helps guide good decisions about epilepsy surgery and can help neurologists localize or confirm the seizure focus. The function of different parts of the brain are very specialized. For example, the medial temporal lobe is important for short-term memory. The temporal lobe on one side of the brain deals more with memory for words and names (verbal), while the other temporal lobe is more specialized for remembering directions and pictures (spatial). If neuropsychological testing shows cognitive problems only in an isolated area, that information may point to the seizure focus. If function is good in an area where surgery is planned, counseling about possible risks of decline in that function after surgery needs to occur. Neuropsychological testing can also provide a baseline assessment that can be used to compare with function after surgery.

Finally, epilepsy surgery is a big undertaking. It is important that doctors identify and addresses any issues with mood or anxiety *before* undergoing a surgical procedure.

In some instances, all of the information from this standard epilepsy surgery evaluation lines up (we say it is **concordant**, meaning in agreement and consistent). If this is the case, epilepsy surgery may be able to be undertaken without any further tests. I introduced Robert at the beginning of this chapter. He was having seizures that did not respond to medications. Imagine if his standard epilepsy surgery evaluation resulted in the following findings:

- His history suggested temporal lobe seizures.
- His MRI showed a right temporal abnormality (right mesial temporal atrophy).
- His interictal EEG showed right temporal spikes.
- His video-EEG study recorded five seizures, all coming from the right temporal lobe.
- His neuropsychological testing showed only difficulties that could be attributed to the right temporal lobe (trouble remembering pictures and diagrams).

If this were the case, he might be able to proceed directly to surgery. In reality, however, things were a little more complicated for Robert. Video-EEG monitoring was not able to detect exactly where the seizures were coming from. This did *not* mean that Robert was excluded as a candidate for epilepsy surgery. It just meant that our standard techniques for doing video-EEG monitoring were not adequate to identify the seizure focus and needed to be supported with other testing. Further exploration could give the answer. Was there more than one seizure focus? Was it simply not possible to find it? Or would additional testing demonstrate convincingly that seizures *were* coming from the suspected right temporal lobe focus?

Advanced Epilepsy Surgery Testing

Several additional diagnostic procedures, introduced in Chapter 7, may be used by the epilepsy surgery team to clarify any questions that remain after a standard epilepsy surgery evaluation. The neurologist and epilepsy surgery team will guide this process, and the exact mix of testing will be fitted to the unique situation. To build on the description of the tests provided in Chapter 7, this section provides additional discussion of ways that a neurologist might use these tests to come to an ultimate conclusion as to whether a patient is an epilepsy surgery candidate.

Positron emission tomography (PET) and single-photon emission computed tomography (SPECT): Both PET and SPECT can help identify a seizure focus when it cannot be identified by MRI. They might also be useful if two or more possible seizure foci have been identified on MRI.

Magnetoencephalography (MEG): This test may be helpful to better locate a possible seizure focus. Often this can guide more detailed EEG testing (see "Intracranial EEG" hereafter). In some centers, MEG is also used to do brain mapping—to locate critical brain areas in and around the seizure focus in order to make surgery as safe as possible.

Functional MRI/Wada/diffusion tensor imaging: Each of these tests is described in Chapter 7. These tests are mostly used to support the safety of a proposed surgery and to locate critical brain functions and pathways so they can be avoided during a planned epilepsy surgery.

Intracranial EEG: Placing electrodes in or on the surface of the brain is often required when the standard evaluation and additional tests do not provide enough information to proceed directly to surgery. If a limited number of possibilities for the seizure focus are found, these can be tested with intracranial electrodes. If a seizure focus lies near areas of critical brain function, the placement of intracranial electrodes to permit brain mapping may also be needed. A large number of possible situations exist in which intracranial monitoring may be used. Among the most common are:

- No focus is identified on MRI, but other tests have narrowed the possibilities to small areas that can be studied with intracranial electrodes.
- Two possible areas of seizure onset have been identified, and intracranial monitoring is used to distinguish which of those areas is in fact the focus.
- The seizure focus lies close to critical brain structures, and it is important to map out the exact borders of the areas of seizure onset and the important brain areas that need to be avoided.

Intracranial monitoring is a more involved process than going directly to epilepsy surgery, and it does carry a small amount of additional risk. However, in some cases it may be the only means of arriving at a successful epilepsy surgery.

Robert did undergo more testing. Because his PET and SPECT scans matched all of the previous testing, with both localizing to the right temporal lobe, his surgery team felt confident that his seizures were coming from that location, and they were able to recommend a right temporal lobe surgery without having to go to intracranial monitoring first. He had no complications with his surgery and has had no seizures since his surgical procedure two years ago.

Surgical Techniques and Alternatives

Most epilepsy surgery is performed as a traditional surgery, in which a portion of the skull is removed, the surgeon sees and surgically removes tissue at the seizure focus, and then closes the skull.

Remarkable advances have been made in the more than 60 years that surgery for epilepsy has been commonly performed. Many of these advancements include improvements in diagnostic testing and refinement of selection of candidates for epilepsy surgery—in other words, finding those people who would benefit from epilepsy surgery and avoiding surgery in those who would not.

Additionally, advances have been made both in the process of surgery itself and in the surrounding support systems to make surgery safer and more effective. Basic advances in anesthesia care, intensive care, and other systems of hospital care have all improved the safety of epilepsy surgery. In the operating room, technical advancements have transformed the process of epilepsy surgery. Computer-guided imaging now frequently supports the epilepsy surgeon. Using an MRI image that has been obtained with location markers, the surgeon can use a probe to touch points on the skull or brain during surgery and view in three-dimensional space the location of the operation relative to the MRI landmarks. This can help the surgeon fully remove an abnormality seen on MRI (making the surgery more effective) and avoid important anatomical areas (making the surgery safer).

After a period of recovery for a few days in the hospital, the healing process continues at home. In is important to know that AED therapy is continued unchanged through the early recovery period after surgery. If a patient remains seizure free, AED treatment can often be simplified to a single medication if more than one has been used or to lower doses of a single AED. Doctors typically will not consider discontinuing AED therapy altogether until after a person has been seizure free for 2 or more years. A substantial number of people who discontinue AEDs even after 2 or more years of seizure freedom still may have late seizure recurrence. Thus epilepsy surgery may not always be a "cure." Rather, it may convert a previously medically refractory epilepsy into one that is relatively easily controlled with low-dose AEDs. For this reason, many people choose to stay on low- or moderate-dose AED monotherapy long term. Please see the section "Epilepsy Surgery Frequently Asked Questions" at the end of this chapter for more comments on some practical aspects of epilepsy surgery. Please note that the details of surgery differ for each individual, and there is no substitute for a detailed discussion with your epilepsy surgery team and epilepsy surgeon about your particular circumstances.

In the temporal lobe, two common and somewhat "standard" procedures are performed. The traditional approach to epilepsy surgery in the temporal lobe is an **anterior temporal lobectomy (ATL)** (Figure 11–2). With this procedure, the surgeon typically removes the anterior (front) 3 to 5 centimeters (1 to 2 inches) of the temporal lobe. This allows access to the deeper, middle part of the temporal lobe, where seizure often begin. The surgery is then completed by removal of these medial temporal lobe structures. Prior to surgery, information about the location of language function is obtained (see "Wada Test" and "Functional Magnetic Resonance Imaging," Chapter 7). The surgery is often modified if it is performed in the temporal lobe that contains language function.

The majority of refractory temporal lobe epilepsy arises from the *medial* temporal lobe. In certain instances, for example in people with mesial temporal sclerosis (MTS), it has been recognized that the ATL procedure probably removes more of the temporal lobe than is necessary to achieve seizure control. Therefore an alternative to ATL was developed, called **selective amygdalohippocampectomy (SAH)** (Figure 11–2). This very long name essentially describes the surgery. It is a selective surgery, in that it targets removal of a limited amount of brain tissue. The targeted areas are in the medial temporal lobe: the hippocampus and the amygdala. These areas are deep in the middle portion of the temporal lobe, and a number of techniques have been developed to selectively target these areas. Much of the temporal lobe normally removed in an ATL is preserved by going under, over, or through the more lateral parts of the temporal lobe. MRI-based computer-guided navigation has made this procedure more feasible and safer. If people with definite

Anterior Temporal Lobectomy   Amygdalohippocampectomy

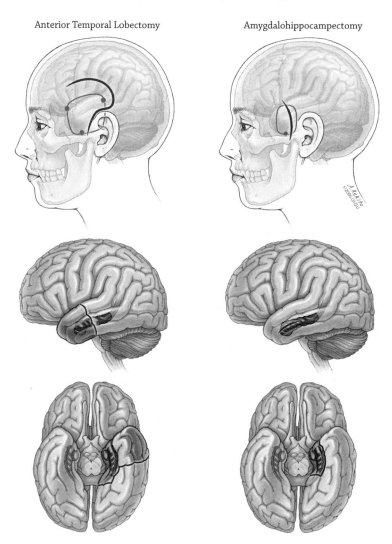

FIGURE 11-2 Anterior temporal lobectomy and selective amygdalohippocampectomy. Images courtesy of Andy Rekito.

medial temporal lobe epilepsy are selected for this procedure, the seizure-free outcomes are very similar to that with ATL. There is some controversy over whether cognitive (thinking) outcomes are superior with the more selective procedure. However, most would agree that less is better when it comes to removing brain tissue that is not directly involved in the seizure focus.

Epilepsy surgery can also be done when the focus is outside of the temporal lobe, but these surgeries are less standard. If an abnormality or "lesion" is seen on MRI that corresponds to the seizure focus, the surgery may consist of removal of that lesion (sometimes called a "lesionectomy"). If there is no visible seizure focus on MRI, the surgery has to be tailored to removal of the focus that is identified by other means, such as EEG.

In recent years, a number of alternatives to traditional open surgery have been explored. The best studied of these is **stereotactic radiosurgery**. Stereotactic radiosurgery is a form of radiation treatment. It uses highly focused beams of radiation coming from different directions to focus on a precise target. It delivers minimal radiation to surrounding normal tissue and has been used to treat tumors and blood vessel abnormalities. Experience is growing with regard to its use to treat temporal lobe epilepsy. The chief advantage of stereotactic radiosurgery is that it is not surgery in the conventional sense. No scalpels are used, and no craniotomy (opening of the skull) is needed. Following planning and calculations based on MRI studies, the treatment can usually be delivered in a single session. This is very attractive compared to undergoing an open surgery. But is it an effective treatment for temporal lobe epilepsy?

The answer is a qualified yes. One notable feature is the delayed response to treatment. With open surgery, an immediate response is usually seen in people who are destined to be seizure free. With stereotactic radiosurgery, the response is substantially delayed. Some seizure types, especially simple partial seizures (auras) may temporarily become *more* difficult to control for a period of time. The area treated with radiosurgery may swell, and this sometimes requires treatment with steroid medications. These changes generally resolve by 2 years post-surgery, at which time the epilepsy outcome can be assessed. Uncertainties still exist regarding the ideal dose of radiation and target. With high-dose treatment, the long-term outcomes approach those of traditional surgery. Some people are attracted to the noninvasive nature of this therapy, while others are hesitant because of the slow response time. The short-term safety profile appears good. Whether there are long-term problems with exposure to radiation therapy remains somewhat uncertain.

Other types of epilepsy may also be considered for stereotactic radiotherapy. These include epilepsy caused by small blood vessel malformations and epilepsy caused by hypothalamic hamartomas, a rare cause that occurs deep in the center of the brain that is difficult to target with conventional surgery. We hope to learn in coming years how this therapy best fits into the range of options for people with medically refractory epilepsy.

Seeing increasing use are laser therapy techniques. Laser therapy allows quicker recovery from surgery, but long-term outcomes are not yet known. More treatment options—especially noninvasive options—would be welcomed, if found to be safe and effective. If you are considering epilepsy surgery, it is a good idea to discuss the full range of options available to you with your neurologist and surgery team.

The Decision to Undergo Epilepsy Surgery

This chapter on epilepsy surgery has covered a lot of ground. We have learned what people are possible candidates for epilepsy surgery and what forms of epilepsy are potentially surgically treatable. We examined the selection and evaluation process for epilepsy surgery and, finally, discussed some of the surgical approaches and techniques that are used.

But if you have medically refractory epilepsy and are in the midst of this process, how should you participate in the decision about whether to go forward with a surgery?

In all cases, the decision making is a partnership between you and your epilepsy surgery team. Nearly all epilepsy surgery is elective. This means that the surgery does not *have* to be done as a lifesaving procedure. It is a choice—a choice to step beyond AED therapy to try to achieve seizure freedom.

Because epilepsy surgery is elective, it means that there is time for you to consider the options and ask questions. Most of the decision making centers on a consideration of the potential *risks* and the potential *benefits* of surgery.

Sometimes the decision making is relatively easy.

After 10 years of medically refractory epilepsy and trials of eight AEDs, Michael underwent an epilepsy surgery evaluation at age 31. Many might argue this evaluation should have been done sooner. His standard epilepsy surgery evaluation showed right mesial temporal sclerosis on MRI scan and multiple seizures recorded on video-EEG, all coming from the right mesial temporal region. His other tests were concordant, and his Wada test showed that language function was located in his other (left) hemisphere, and that his left temporal lobe memory function was good. His chances of seizure freedom with surgery were felt to be high, and the risk of surgery low. He chose to go forward with surgery and has been seizure free for the last 5 years.

Decision making for Deven was also relatively easy.

Deven was thought to have lateral temporal lobe epilepsy based on standard epilepsy surgery testing and some additional specialized imaging studies. His MRI was normal, but his epilepsy team felt confident that a region of seizure onset was identified. They proposed that intracranial monitoring be done to pinpoint the area of seizure onset. He agreed to go forward,

(Continued)

(*Continued*)

and the neurosurgeon placed a large grid array of electrodes over the area of suspected seizure onset. Unfortunately, when seizures were recorded, it was not possible to locate the area of seizure onset. The entire grid appeared to show onset at the same time, and despite specialized analysis of the recordings, it was not possible to locate the zone of seizure onset. The epilepsy surgery team advised him that it was best to simply remove the grids and not attempt a surgery to remove a seizure focus. Such a surgery would be a "shot in the dark." It would be unlikely to provide better seizure control and would carry the potential to cause new deficits.

Other times, decision making can enter a gray area, where there is no absolute right or wrong thing to do. It is in these situations that the partnership for decision making between the patient and the epilepsy surgery team is especially important. Many situations can be imagined, but here are a couple of "real world" examples.

Tania has occipital lobe epilepsy. She had cancer as a child and had to undergo chemotherapy that affected her immune system. She developed a brain abscess—a localized brain infection—in the occipital lobe that had to be treated with antibiotics and surgical drainage. She is now 35 and free of cancer, but she has had refractory focal epilepsy for years. Her standard epilepsy surgery evaluation and some specialized imaging studies pointed to the area of injury in the occipital lobe. She underwent intracranial monitoring to more precisely map out the area of onset relative to areas important for visual function in the region. The epilepsy team localized her

(*Continued*)

(*Continued*)

seizures using the grid, but the seizures arose from a region that partly overlapped with areas important for visual function. If the entire region was removed, she would certainly have visual loss—possibly for half of her visual field. If the surgery were more limited, it would preserve visual function but would be less likely to result in complete seizure freedom. The epilepsy team did not simply ask Tania what surgery she wanted to have. Rather, they laid out the facts, answered questions, and had some difficult back-and-forth discussions to find out how Tania, her husband, and her family felt about the choices. Ultimately Tania felt that being seizure free but impaired and unable to drive because of visual problems would not be a good tradeoff. A more limited surgery was performed. Tania recovered with full visual function and no other new problems. Her seizures are better—much better—but not gone. Previously she had several seizures per month. Now, she has a breakthrough seizure about every 2 to 3 months and is exploring some new AED options.

Carlos was 43 and had medically refractory temporal lobe epilepsy. His MRI suggested mesial temporal sclerosis on the left. During video-EEG monitoring, nine seizures were recorded. Eight of these were typical seizures. He had his typical aura, and his family recognized the typical sequence of events that followed. All eight of these came from the left temporal lobe. However, he had interictal epileptiform discharges (sharp waves) in both temporal lobes (left more than right), and during sleep one seizure was recorded with onset in the *right*

(*Continued*)

(*Continued*)

temporal lobe. The general rule for epilepsy surgery is that a single seizure focus must be identified. This allows the best chances of seizure freedom—the goal of most epilepsy surgery. If half of his typical seizures had come from each side, he would not usually be considered a surgical candidate. But in this case, Carlos's epilepsy surgery team did feel like they could potentially offer surgery on the left temporal lobe, but with the caution that although it might help make his seizures more manageable, they had reduced expectations for seizure freedom. The risks and benefits were clearly different from someone whose testing was all concordant in identifying a single focus. The decision making was difficult, but he elected to go forward with surgery and fortunately did very well. He had no new difficulties with function after his surgery, and after 3 years he was seizure free. His neurologist has advised against attempting to decrease his seizure medication because the risk of seizures recurring off of AEDs was felt to be relatively high.

At the heart of every decision is a balancing of the risks and benefits. In general, the odds are best with mesial temporal sclerosis and concordant test findings. Odds of seizure freedom are also quite good with an MRI-identified seizure focus and concordant testing. In some cases, although success rates may decline with surgical treatment of epilepsy outside of the temporal lobe, they may still be very good. If seizures begin outside the temporal lobe *and* there is no MRI abnormality, the chances of seizure freedom are even lower. But this is just talking about general groups of patients. If you are undergoing epilepsy surgery evaluation, you may have a specific finding on MRI, in a specific location, along with a particular EEG pattern and a unique description of your seizure symptoms. Your epilepsy surgery team will do their best to give at least approximate odds of seizure freedom following a proposed surgery so that you can understand the "benefit" side of the equation.

What about risk? All surgical procedures can have risks, and epilepsy surgery is no exception. Your epilepsy surgery team, including your neurosurgeon, will discuss the risks specific to any surgery that might be considered. You might consider and ask about risks in two categories:

1. General risks of neurosurgical procedures: These include risks of anesthesia (generally very small) and risks of unexpected complications such as bleeding, stroke (blockage of blood flow to a part of the brain), and infection. Your epilepsy surgery team or neurosurgeon will discuss these risks with you. For most epilepsy surgery procedures these risks are relatively small, in the neighborhood of 1 to 2 percent risk. Of course, if you are in that 1 or 2 percent, it can be very serious, so it is worth consideration. The risk of death from a surgical procedure is always discussed, but with epilepsy surgery the risk is extraordinarily low.

2. Risks specific to the surgical procedure being considered: Beyond the general risks of neurosurgery, there may be some risks specific to a surgery you might be considering. Often these risks relate to the brain functions located close to the seizure focus. These are unique for each person and cannot all be discussed here. You should ask your epilepsy surgery team if there are any unique risks with any surgery being proposed for you. These risks could come from blood vessels in the area of the planned surgery, unique brain functions located near the surgery site, or from other medical conditions that you might have.

If you are undergoing one of the more "standard" temporal lobe surgeries previously discussed (ATL or SAH), some common potential risks are usually discussed. Some language function is located in the temporal lobe, so if an operation is being considered in the temporal lobe that contains language function, it is good to ask about any possible risks to language function. Modification of an ATL, or doing the more focused SAH, procedure may minimize this risk.

One of the main functions of the medial temporal lobe is short-term memory, and potential risks to memory, if any, need to be understood and discussed.

In some cases, especially when temporal lobe epilepsy begins early in life, some of the normal function for short-term memory at the seizure focus is shifted to other parts of the brain. The affected part of the brain (the seizure focus) may not be contributing much to memory function, and in fact the intermittent seizures may disrupt the function of neighboring brain regions. In situations like this, the risk to memory function from surgery may be small. In some instances, improvement in some aspects of memory function may be seen if seizures are effectively stopped and neighboring regions are able to function better without the disturbances of intermittent seizures. However, the expectation should not be that epilepsy surgery will improve memory function. If the seizures can be stopped and memory function remains unchanged or minimally affected, that is usually considered a good outcome.

In some people, a greater risk of worsening memory following temporal lobe surgery can be predicted. The risk is greater in people who had seizure onset later in life, probably because they are less able than children to shift function to other brain regions. Those who have a normal-appearing hippocampus on MRI, those whose memory function is excellent prior to surgery, and those who are having surgery on the temporal lobe that contains language function are all at somewhat greater risk of memory problems after surgery. All of these factors predict that there might be "more to lose" with respect to short-term memory. An assessment of these factors, often combined with results from a Wada test, can be used for counseling about any potential risks to short-term memory prior to making a decision about surgery. If a surgery would be likely to cause severe memory problems, it is generally not offered as an option.

The temporal lobe has limited involvement with vision, but some of the visual pathways (the "wires") that connect the eyes to the visual areas in the back of the brain pass through the temporal lobe. Thus temporal lobe surgery (both ATL and SAH) can potentially affect vision in a limited way. If these pathways are disrupted by surgery, affected persons can develop what is called a visual field defect. Almost always, these individuals are unaware of a change in their vision. They do not see a "black spot" or notice anything missing in their visual world. But if they focus on a spot, and an object is shown in their peripheral vision ("side vision") up high on the side opposite where the surgery was done, they may not be able to see the object. If they shift their vision to look directly at the object, they can see it normally. This visual field deficit is sometimes called a "pie in the sky," because a pie-shaped wedge of peripheral vision in the upper vision, opposite from the side of surgery, is affected. This same area can be found in both eyes if tested individually. The risk differs somewhat by type and extent of procedure. A "pie in the sky" defect is identified in one-third of people undergoing temporal lobe epilepsy surgery, and with detailed testing more subtle defects appear to be very common. Usually mild visual field defects in this area don't affect daily function.

Finally, the medial temporal lobe is also part of the circuits that regulate emotions. Mood disturbances are common in epilepsy. In some people, epilepsy surgery can worsen mood or increase anxiety, at least in the short-term. If you have been struggling with anxiety or depression, it is important to identify and treat this before surgery. After surgery, it is also wise for you and your family and friends to be alert to the possibility of worsening mood or anxiety so that it can be identified early and effectively treated.

In sum, epilepsy surgery can be a highly effective treatment and can often provide the opportunity for seizure freedom in people who were not substantially helped by AED therapy. The process starts with identification of medically refractory epilepsy and an epilepsy syndrome that is surgically treatable. A standard, or at times expanded, epilepsy surgery evaluation provides the basis for understanding the potential risks and benefits of surgery and guides decision making.

The prospect of brain surgery can be scary. Feeling frightened to contemplate it is a normal response. However, the limited risks of epilepsy surgery need to be balanced with *the risk of doing nothing*. Medically refractory epilepsy is also risky. It carries risk of injury, prolonged disability, and a higher risk of sudden death than the general population as a result of uncontrolled seizures. Some evidence shows that successful epilepsy surgery can markedly reduce the risk of sudden death from poorly controlled seizures. Many years of poorly controlled seizures can affect cognition (thinking and memory). Finally, epilepsy and epilepsy surgery are not all about counting seizures. The point is really about quality of life, and several studies show marked improvement in quality of life in people who have effective epilepsy surgery.

Epilepsy Surgery Frequently Asked Questions

How long does an epilepsy surgery procedure last?

The length of an epilepsy surgery can vary a great deal depending on the procedure and the necessary preparation and recovery time. Many epilepsy surgeries take somewhere between 2 and 4 hours. Your surgeon or neurologist will be able to give you more specific information for your case.

How long will I need to be in the hospital?

This also can vary greatly depending on the procedure and the practices of your surgery team. At many centers patients are closely observed in the intensive care unit (ICU) overnight following the procedure. Patients are then often moved to a regular hospital bed, usually for another 2 to 4 days, before going home. Your health care team would need to make sure you are eating well, able to walk short distances, and do not require any intravenous (IV) medications before sending you home.

How long is the full recovery period after epilepsy surgery?

The recovery time can also vary depending on the procedure and the person. Many centers advise people to allow 6 weeks of recovery time before resuming full work or other duties. Much of this time involves simply getting full energy and endurance back. It is often helpful to have family members available to help at home, especially for the first 1 to 2 weeks. Surgeons will have specific advice about limitations on lifting and wound care.

Will my whole head be shaved?

Generally it is necessary to shave hair in the region of the surgery, and your health care team can advise you on the area where this would be needed. It is not necessary to shave the entire head, and the hair should grow back normally in the shaved area.

Do you have to remove bone to do the surgery, or do you use a laser?

Most epilepsy surgery is done as an open surgery that involves a craniotomy (removal of skull bone over the site of the surgery), followed by surgical removal of the seizure focus. The surgeon then generally replaces and attaches the bone, which should heal to form a strong protective covering for the brain. New techniques are being developed that are less invasive. Some of these are discussed in this chapter. You can ask your epilepsy surgery team if any of these are appropriate for you.

Will I still have to take medication after the surgery?

Yes, most patients require antiepileptic medication following surgery to remain seizure free. Often the number of antiepileptic medications and dosages can be reduced if you are stable and seizure free for some months following surgery, and some patients who become seizure free for a prolonged period may not require any long-term medication. However, as many as half of people who come off AEDs entirely may ultimately have a late return of a seizure or seizures. Your neurologist will discuss this with you further.

Can epilepsy surgery make a scar on my brain that could cause more seizures?

No, epilepsy surgery does not create a new seizure focus.

What are the chances that the epilepsy surgery will make me seizure free?

This is an individual assessment based on the preoperative testing you have undergone and other factors about your epilepsy that your neurologist will consider. Your neurologist may be able to give you an estimate of the chances of becoming seizure free in your individual situation.

Are there any risks to epilepsy surgery?

All surgical procedures have some risk. The general risks of surgery include bleeding, infection, and increased neurological deficit. The epilepsy team will not offer surgery if it appears to be excessively risky. Your neurologist and neurosurgeon will discuss the potential surgical risks with you prior to any surgery.

Will I be awake during the surgery?

Nearly all epilepsy surgery is done with the patient asleep. In rare instances, portions of the surgery are done with the patient awake to map critical brain areas, with medications given to prevent pain. Your doctor will tell you if this more rare procedure is needed in your case.

Chapter 12

Beyond AEDs

Other Therapeutic Options

Nearly everyone with epilepsy is treated with some form of anti-epileptic medication. When medications are not working, early evaluation for epilepsy surgery is advised. If standard medication is not working, and you are not a candidate for epilepsy surgery or choose to not undergo surgery, what other alternatives do you have? Fortunately, other good options exist. This chapter explores additional treatments for epilepsy, including neurostimulation, complementary and alternative medicine, and diet therapy.

Neurostimulation: Medical Devices to Treat Epilepsy

We have learned that antiepileptic drug (AED) therapy can provide seizure freedom for nearly two-thirds of patients with epilepsy. For the remaining one-third, an early assessment for possible epilepsy surgery is strongly recommended. As we have seen, surgical removal of the seizure focus can be both safe and highly effective in selected individuals.

But what if you are not a candidate for surgery? This is a situation that confronts many people. As previously suggested, there are many possible reasons why a person might not be a candidate for epilepsy surgery, including the following:

- Having generalized epilepsy with no single seizure focus to target
- Having focal epilepsy with two or more areas of seizure onset.
- Having focal epilepsy that cannot be adequately localized to allow surgical treatment.
- Having a seizure focus that is in or near critical brain areas where complete removal is not possible.

If you have medically refractory epilepsy and are not a surgical candidate, more choices are available than simply trying additional AEDs. The field of neurostimulation has emerged to fill some of this need. The various forms of neurostimulation for epilepsy will be discussed here. With neurostimulation, therapy is delivered in the form of electrical stimulation to a nerve outside of the brain or to the brain itself. Some forms of neurostimulation require surgery to implant a device, but none are "epilepsy surgery" in the traditional sense—the surgery is simply to place the device, and no brain tissue is removed. While none of these forms of neurostimulation is as effective as epilepsy surgery—most have only a very small chance of producing seizure freedom—as a group they represent a different way of delivering therapy that can work together with AEDs to move closer to the goal of seizure freedom.

Vagus Nerve Stimulation

Vagus nerve stimulation (**VNS**) was the first form of neurostimulation approved for the treatment of epilepsy, in 1997. With VNS, a pacemaker-like device (Figure 12–1) is implanted in the chest that delivers electrical stimulation to a nerve in the neck called the vagus nerve. Since 1997, more than 100,000 people have received VNS therapy. The official approval for the device is for adjunctive (add-on) treatment of medically refractory focal epilepsy in people over 12 years of age. Generally these are people who are not candidates for epilepsy surgery to remove the seizure focus. VNS therapy has

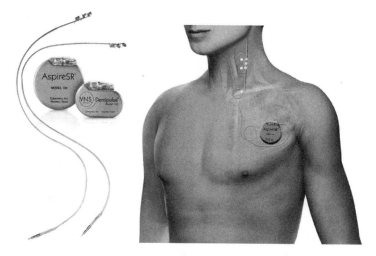

FIGURE 12-1 Vagus Nerve Stimulator. Images courtesy of Cyberonics, Inc.

been used "**off label**" (outside of the standard approvals) beyond this described group. Use in children has been fairly common, and a recent review of all available evidence concluded cautiously that it is "possibly effective" in children, although it has not been approved by the US Food and Drug Administration (FDA) for this group. The device has also been used off label for people with other epilepsy syndromes, such as Lennox-Gastaut syndrome, and there is evidence that it is "possibly effective" in these groups, as well.

The vagus nerve is one of the 12 pairs of cranial nerves in the head and neck. Both the left and right vagus nerves pass through the neck as they connect areas near the base of the brain (the brainstem) to different parts of the body. The vagus nerve helps carry signals that control some basic functions. These include signals to the stomach, lungs, heart, and larynx ("voice box"). By a process that is still not well understood, it was found that electrical stimulation of the vagus nerve could send signals to the brainstem, which has many connections to the cortex, where seizures are generated.

Research showed that these signals to the cortex decreased the likelihood of seizures in animals. A similar effect was later proven in people with epilepsy.

Those receiving VNS therapy first undergo a relatively simple procedure to place the device. The device is usually implanted under general anesthesia (people are "asleep" for the procedure). A pacemaker-like device, called a generator, is placed by a surgeon under the skin on the left side of the chest. During the same procedure, a wire or "lead" is gently wrapped around the left vagus nerve in the neck, passed under the skin, and connected to the generator. This requires two surgical openings or incisions—one in the upper chest and one in the neck. The procedure is usually a day surgery with no overnight stay in the hospital. Recovery at home is usually fairly quick, and within a few weeks, stimulation therapy can begin. Depending on the settings, the battery in the generator may last 5 to 7 years or more. At the end of battery life, a more minor surgical procedure is required to replace the generator if VNS therapy is to continue.

Once the implant is in place, doctors can program the VNS generator in the clinic by the use of a handheld computer and a "wand." The wand is a flat plastic device that is placed on the skin overlying the generator. This allows the programmer to "talk" to the device and change settings. The device is programmed for intermittent stimulation. Typical starting settings are 30 seconds of stimulation on followed by 5 minutes off. This programming is set so that the device goes off and on by itself, 24 hours a day, 7 days a week. Doctors can change a number of different settings to find those that best control seizures. Changes are usually made over a period of weeks as the "dose" of stimulation is gradually adjusted. Sometimes more frequent bursts of stimulation ("rapid cycling") have been tried to obtain better seizure control, although there is no strong evidence that this works better.

The device has another interesting feature: You have some control over the device! After implantation, individuals receive a magnet that can be carried or worn on the wrist; alternatively, a family member or caregiver can carry the magnet. The magnet has two uses.

First, it can be used to trigger a cycle of stimulation "on demand"—when it is needed at the start of a seizure. This is especially useful for people who have an aura before their seizures. The magnet can be passed over the device for a few seconds to trigger stimulation when an aura is felt. For some people, this stimulation may prevent the seizure from progressing. At other times it might result in a milder seizure or lead to more rapid recovery. If you don't have an aura before your seizures, don't worry—this is not required to see benefit from use of the VNS.

Second, the magnet can be used to temporarily "turn off," or disable, the device. If the magnet is placed over the generator *and kept there*, it will temporarily shut off the VNS device as long as the magnet stays there. This can be reassuring for people who live far away from their doctor, in the unlikely event that they have concerns about the function of the device or if they are experiencing any discomfort. The magnet can be held in place with a piece of tape to turn off the device until it can be checked. Once the magnet is removed, the device resumes its regular cycles.

When I reviewed decision making for epilepsy surgery, I talked about assessing risks and benefits. The same goes for a decision to pursue VNS therapy. While it is not a brain surgery, it is still a big step, and a commitment to have a device implanted.

First, the potential benefits. The best evidence comes from the carefully conducted randomized controlled studies that led to the approval of the device. These studies suggested that seizures were reduced by nearly one-third, on average, over the short course of the study. About one-third of people with the device were considered to be responders to the therapy. A "responder" is someone whose usual number of seizures was reduced by at least half. Several attempts were made to look at longer-term outcome after a year or more of therapy. These results are harder to interpret because they are "open label." This means that there was no longer a placebo comparison group. Also, other changes such as AED adjustments could be made. The best of these studies suggested improved responses over time, with seizures reduced by nearly 50 percent on average by 1 year. As with several forms of neurostimulation, the benefits appear to increase over time.

The main benefits of VNS therapy are on epilepsy. However, a secondary consideration can be positive effects on mood. The VNS is also approved for treatment of treatment-resistant depression (a separate use of the device). A recent review of the use of VNS for epilepsy found evidence that it is possibly effective for reducing depression and improving mood. However, this should not be the main reason for VNS implantation in someone with epilepsy, and it does not replace traditional medical and talk therapy for depression.

What was also apparent from the studies was that becoming seizure free on VNS therapy was exceedingly rare. In all of these studies, VNS therapy was added to, and did not replace, AED therapy.

What about the risks? VNS implantation requires surgery. There are general risks of going under anesthesia and from the implant procedure, but these are quite small. In studies, the risk of infection was about 1.5 percent. That means a little more than 1 person in 100 had this problem. If used off label in children, the infection rate is higher and must be watched carefully. An infection could create a need to remove the entire VNS implant. Although the vagus nerve has connections to several organ systems, including the heart, problems with heart rhythm disturbances from stimulation have been carefully looked for and are rare. Injury to the vagus nerve can occur in up to 1 in 100 implants. If this happens, it can cause paralysis of one of the vocal cords, leading to hoarseness and possibly swallowing problems. All of these risks are small. The most common side effect of VNS is hoarseness or coughing as a result of the intermittent stimulation. If the strength of the stimulation is increased too rapidly, stimulation can be painful and hoarseness and coughing can be prominent. There is no evidence that rapidly increasing stimulation provides any benefit. Thus it is important to make changes slowly. VNS therapy should not be a painful experience. However, even with slow increases in stimulation, a change in the quality of the voice may occur during stimulation. It may sound "hoarse," "coarse," or "gravelly." This tends to resolve over time but may reappear if the strength of the VNS settings is increased. If voice changes cause difficulties at certain times, the magnet can be used to temporarily disable the VNS. Some of my patients will tape the magnet over their device when they do public speaking. Another of my patients sings in the church choir and uses the magnet to turn off the device during rehearsals and performances.

Importantly, VNS side effects are quite different from side effects produced by AEDs. If you have tried many different AEDs, you may be relieved to hear that VNS therapy is not expected to cause dizziness, drowsiness, slowed thinking, or other typical AED side effects. One additional limitation of VNS therapy relates to MRI scans. Once the device is implanted, it is not safe to do an MRI scan of the chest and abdomen, as the device or the lead might heat up, causing injury. With proper precautions, an MRI scan of the brain can be safely performed. Use of household appliances such as microwave ovens, hair dryers, and cellphones will not affect the function of the VNS device. Those with VNS devices receive ID cards that can be used to notify airport screeners.

VNS therapy can be considered in many people older than age 12 with medically refractory focal epilepsy who are not candidates for epilepsy surgery. If epilepsy surgery is possible, it is usually preferred, as it is much more likely to produce complete seizure freedom. Some doctors may consider VNS therapy for children and people who do not have focal epilepsy, but this use is considered off label—not wrong, but not officially sanctioned by the FDA. Many experts recommend performing video-EEG monitoring prior to VNS implant. This could serve to confirm that the individual is not a candidate for curative epilepsy surgery. It can also confirm the epilepsy diagnosis. A VNS device should not be implanted in someone who has nonepileptic events.

Responsive Neurostimulation

Responsive neurostimulation (RNS) is the latest entry into the field of neurostimulation treatments for epilepsy. The concept of RNS is different from VNS in several ways.

First, instead of more distant stimulation of a nerve in the neck, the electrical stimulation with RNS therapy is delivered directly to the seizure focus. Second, instead of delivering intermittent stimulation on a fixed schedule, the stimulation is *responsive*. This means it is only delivered when the very beginning of a seizure is detected. Otherwise the device remains at rest. How is this possible?

First, some brief background. For years it had been noted that delivery of a small electrical stimulation to a seizure focus could sometimes abort (stop) a developing seizure. It was not until recently that technology caught up with this concept, and development of a miniaturized device that could detect seizures and deliver stimulation back to the focus became possible. Those advances in technology paved the way for the NeuroPace® RNS® System.

The RNS System includes the RNS generator and two leads (Figure 12–2). These leads could be depth electrodes (thin spears that go into the brain near the seizure focus) or strip electrodes (small, flat disks embedded in a flexible plastic strip that sits on the surface of the brain at the seizure focus). These leads are connected to the generator, which contains a battery and small computer. The entire system is placed in the head by a neurosurgeon. The leads go in or on the seizure focus, and the generator replaces a small piece of skull and lies flat with the rest of the skull—there is no visible bump. When this device is in place, it constantly monitors electrical activity recorded at the leads. When a pattern that represents that individual's seizures is seen, the device responds rapidly with a burst

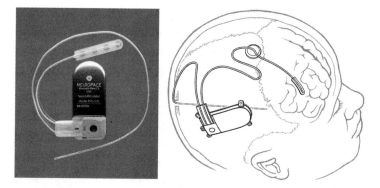

FIGURE 12–2 NeuroPace® RNS® System. Images courtesy of NeuroPace, Inc.

of electrical stimulation to the seizure focus. The goal is to disrupt the developing seizure before it produces any symptoms. The electrical stimulation cannot be felt. With the use of a laptop and a "wand" that is placed on the head over the device, the patient or a caregiver can transmit EEG recordings from the device to a secure website. The treating provider can then view the EEG activity, including seizures. Over time, the device can be taught how to better recognize that person's seizures early, and the best settings for the responsive stimulation can be determined.

After early studies of the device showed a good safety profile, a larger study was undertaken to demonstrate the effectiveness of the device in a larger group of adults with very-difficult-to-control focal epilepsy. After a period of observation, half of the people who had the device implanted had it turned on, and half received "sham" stimulation for the first 12 weeks. Sham stimulation means that the researchers went through the motions as if they were programming the device, but they did not turn it on. After 12 weeks *everyone* had stimulation turned on and received the benefits of therapy. This allowed a very scientific evaluation of the effectiveness of RNS therapy.

The trial clearly showed that active therapy worked better than sham therapy, and the device was approved by the FDA in November 2013. In this short study, the average percent reduction in seizures at the end of the 12-week comparison period was nearly 40 percent. When people were followed on therapy for a longer period of time, the results improved. The average percent seizure reduction was 44 percent at 1 year, and 53 percent at 2 years. At long-term follow-up about 15 percent of this group with very-difficult-to-control seizures was seizure free for at least 6 months.

That gives an idea of the potential benefit, but what about the risks? The device met the FDA's safety measures. It appeared at least as safe as a previously approved device for deep brain stimulation for Parkinson's disease. Implantation does carry all the potential risks of surgery, including risks of infection and bleeding. Small numbers of both of these events were seen in the studies. The stimulation itself appeared safe, and no negative effects (and possibly some positive ones) were seen on mood, cognition, and quality of life.

Only a highly select group of people are candidates for RNS therapy. The system is approved for use in adults; the device has not yet been studied in children. It is specifically approved for use in medically refractory focal epilepsy where diagnostic testing has localized one or two seizure foci. Localization of the seizure focus is a very important issue. While VNS can be used without knowing the location of the seizure focus, this localization is critical for effective use of RNS. As with other forms of neurostimulation, RNS therapy is not usually preferred if a safe and effective epilepsy surgery option is available. In this situation, epilepsy surgery is much more likely to result in seizure freedom. Because the two RNS leads can be placed in different parts of the brain, it *can* be used to treat people who are not surgical candidates because they have two seizure-onset zones. It could also be an attractive option for people in whom the seizure focus is known, but nearby important brain structures make surgical removal of the focus unsafe. Implant of the RNS device makes it difficult to perform some brain imaging tests, so RNS therapy is not recommended for anyone with a progressive brain condition such as a brain tumor that might require monitoring with neuroimaging.

RNS therapy may be a very attractive option for people with well-localized focal epilepsy who, for various reasons, cannot undergo epilepsy surgery. The concept of monitoring electrical activity and stimulating, instead of removing, brain tissue is very appealing. Solid evidence of its benefit exists, and further experience will help to determine the ideal candidates for this therapy and the optimal detection and stimulation settings.

Other Forms of Neurostimulation

The field of neurostimulation research is very active. A large trial of another form of stimulation, called **deep brain stimulation (DBS)**, was recently performed. DBS for epilepsy is similar to the DBS used to treat Parkinson's disease, which many people have heard of. However, for epilepsy, a different target deep in the brain, called the anterior nucleus of the thalamus, was used. The study was successfully completed with some positive findings, but it was not approved for use by the FDA because they determined that the evidence for effectiveness was not convincing enough. It has been approved for use in some other countries.

Stimulation of other nerves is also being investigated. Advanced studies have been performed on an external stimulator of another one of the cranial nerves, called the trigeminal nerve. This approach is unique because there is no surgery. The electrode is applied to the skin on the forehead and provides stimulation during sleep and while doing quiet activities at home. Early results have generated interest, and larger studies in people with epilepsy are ongoing.

Complementary and Alternative Medicine in Epilepsy

The term "complementary and alternative medicine" (CAM) refers to forms of therapy that are outside of the mainstream of conventional medicine. Technically, complementary therapy describes those alternative practices that are used *together* with conventional medicine. Alternative therapies are those used *in place of* conventional Western medicine. Here they will be considered together as CAM therapy.

Mitchell is 49 years old and has had epilepsy for 3 years, following a traumatic brain injury from a motor vehicle accident. The injury also affected Mitchell's thinking and memory, although these problems have improved substantially since his accident and have now stabilized. His seizures are nearly completely controlled on carbamazepine (Tegretol). He still experiences about one breakthrough seizure per year, sometimes related to forgetting a dose of his carbamazepine. He often feels tired, and his thinking is slower than he would like. He attributes both of these symptoms to treatment with carbamazepine. Once he ran out of medications for 2 days, and he felt that his thinking was much clearer; however he then experienced one of his most severe generalized tonic-clonic seizures and immediately went back on carbamazepine.

Mitchell's friend told him about an herbal supplement that might help with his seizures. The idea that this was "natural" appealed to Mitchell. He did more reading on the Internet and also found information about herbal supplements that might help with his memory. Mitchell had a good relationship with his doctor and shared this information with her at their next visit.

Mitchell is not alone in his interest in CAM therapy. The numbers vary by region and population, but several studies suggest that at least one-third of people with epilepsy in the United States use CAM therapy. Their reasons for use are many. First, CAM therapies tend to be more popular in conditions where conventional medicine is incompletely effective. Given that at least one-third of people with epilepsy fail to get adequate control with conventional medicine, there is a large group who might want to explore alternatives. Some people may have difficulty getting access to conventional medicine, although this is slowly improving. People with epilepsy may have other related health issues, and CAM therapy is often directed at these other problems. These could include mood problems, such as anxiety or depression. Sleep can be affected. Memory concerns are often at the forefront. In some cases, AEDs may be effective in controlling seizures but carry with them mild or moderate side effects. They may not be bad enough to warrant stopping the AED, but people may seek CAM therapy to help manage these side effects. In some cases, CAM therapy is sought as a more "natural" alternative. In others, it may be in line with cultural practices and beliefs.

Whatever the reason, the use of CAM therapy is widespread. I have mentioned herbal or botanical therapies, but the spectrum of CAM therapies is much broader. It includes homeopathy, acupuncture, mind–body therapies (for example, meditation, yoga, and biofeedback), vitamin therapy, diets, and traditional Chinese medicine and Ayurvedic medicine.

Careful scientific studies of some of these areas have been sparse, despite their widespread use. Comprehensive scientific reviews have been performed in several areas of CAM therapy for epilepsy, including with acupuncture, yoga, and vitamins, and none was able to establish clear evidence of effectiveness.

Of the literally hundreds of herbal CAM therapies in reported use worldwide, those most commonly used in people with epilepsy in the United States (either to treat seizures or, commonly, other associated conditions) include ginseng, St. John's wort, melatonin, ginkgo biloba, garlic, black cohosh, soy, kava kava, and valerian. One particularly controversial area is the use of marijuana, or marijuana extracts, for treatment of epilepsy (for more information on this topic, see the Debates in Epilepsy section in this chapter).

Some people think "natural" CAM therapy means "safe," but that is not always the case. CAM therapy, like any treatment, can also carry risk.

One risk can come with the use of *alternative* therapies—specifically, discontinuing conventional treatment in favor of an alternative and more natural course of treatment. In almost all cases, this cannot be recommended. There can be substantial risk to stopping conventional seizure medication, including safety concerns that can come with having more seizures, the risk of more intense or dangerously prolonged seizures (status epilepticus), and even the potential for **sudden unexpected death in epilepsy (SUDEP)** (see Chapter 3 for a detailed discussion of SUDEP).

Another area of possible concern is interaction of CAM therapies with conventional medications. We already know that many conventional AEDs are prone to interact with other medications. They can also interact with CAM therapies. Much more needs to be understood about potential interactions between the many CAM therapies used and conventional medicine. Several commonly used CAM therapies affect liver systems used in AED metabolism. These include St. John's wort, echinacea, milk thistle, and ginkgo biloba, among others.

Finally, some CAM therapies have the potential to cause or worsen seizures. Among these, black cohosh, kava kava, and ginkgo seeds have been reported to cause seizures. Especially of concern are stimulants that might be included in energy or weight loss preparations. One of these, ephedra, is perhaps the most notorious. In the United States, ephedra temporarily had required warnings and was banned for a period of time. But regulation of herbal therapies falls under "dietary supplements" and is less tightly regulated than pharmaceuticals.

Regulation of Herbal Treatments and Dietary Supplements

Herbals and dietary supplements are not as tightly regulated by the FDA as standard drugs. The main law that guides their marketing and use was passed in 1994. Their producers are restricted from making claims of effectiveness for specific medical conditions. They must follow rules for labeling. They are required to register manufacturing facilities with the FDA and follow good manufacturing practices, but the FDA does not review or approve supplements before they are marketed. A manufacturer does not need to provide evidence of safety and effectiveness to the FDA before marketing a product. Still, they must record, forward to the FDA, and investigate serious problems that are reported to them. The FDA does not routinely analyze products to ensure that the label accurately reflects the ingredients in the product—that burden falls on the manufacturer. Some independent reports have suggested wide variations in the amount of active ingredient that is present in some marketed products. The FDA recommends that concerned consumers contact the manufacturer or a commercial laboratory for an analysis of the content.

It is very helpful that Mitchell had a good relationship with his doctor and that he felt comfortable discussing his planned use of CAM therapy in advance. Unfortunately, many people do not share this important information with their doctor. I would encourage anyone reading this book to bring the use of any CAM therapy to the attention of your doctor. If you have any information about the therapy you are using, bring it along to your clinic visit. Connect your doctor with your naturopathic doctor or other provider who might be recommending your CAM therapy. The range of CAM therapies is quite large, and your provider may not be familiar with the specific approach or product that you are using. Often the education process is a two-way street.

Scientific support for CAM therapy is lacking in many cases. Lack of evidence for benefit does *not* mean that they do not work.

In many cases, it just means that the therapy has not been fully investigated. Clearly, we still need to learn more about which CAM therapies are most effective in epilepsy (and which might be harmful). In this respect, the future is bright. In addition to the work of individual scientists and doctors, the National Center for Complementary and Integrative Health (NCCIH; formerly the National Center for Complementary and Alternative Medicine) was established in 1998. This branch of the National Institutes of Health (NIH) has an annual operating budget of over $100 million and is carrying the study of CAM therapy in many areas to the next level.

Debates in Epilepsy: Epilepsy and Marijuana

Many states with medical marijuana laws include treatment of epilepsy as one of the many permissible reasons for medical marijuana use. But the issue of marijuana and epilepsy hit the popular media in a big way in 2013 when multiple media outlets—including Dr. Sanjay Gupta at CNN—profiled the story of Charlotte Figi. Charlotte's severe childhood epilepsy was poorly controlled despite extensive AED and diet therapy. After much investigation, her parents started her on a marijuana extract, with reported dramatic results. This almost singlehandedly triggered a resurgence of interest in marijuana for the treatment of epilepsy.

Marijuana is not a single substance but rather contains many active ingredients, including about 80 compounds called cannabinoids, as well as hundreds of other compounds. One cannabinoid called THC is the main psychoactive substance (the major contributor to the "high" of marijuana).

(Continued)

(*Continued*)

Cannabidiol (CBD) is another main substance that does not produce a "high" but has multiple actions in the body and brain. Charlotte's parents used a form of marijuana extract that had much more cannabidiol than THC.

Following these and other news reports, marijuana therapy for epilepsy has been rapidly adopted, often with strains thought to be high in CBD, for treatment of both children and adults with epilepsy. There are several reasons why this remains a "hot" and controversial topic.

Many in the medical community have expressed concern that we don't know enough about the safety and effectiveness of these preparations. The scientific data on effectiveness are scant. Animal studies have demonstrated antiepileptic properties of THC, although in some species this same compound may make seizures more likely to occur. Studies of CBD have more consistently suggested an antiepileptic effect.

Sound scientific studies of marijuana or its components in humans are extremely limited. A 2014 review by researchers working with the American Academy of Neurology found no high-quality scientific studies in humans and concluded that there was insufficient data to support its use. In the absence of good scientific studies, there is a risk that placebo effects or selective reporting of successes can make ineffective or even harmful treatments appear helpful. There are many previous examples of this problem where a highly promoted therapy fell into disuse after more scientific information became available. For instance, careful scientific studies altered the practice of prescribing hormone replacement therapy in women. People in difficult or even desperate circumstances may be especially vulnerable to being persuaded to try unproven treatments, as was the experience with the proposed cancer drug Laetrile in

(*Continued*)

(*Continued*)

the 1960s and unproven forms of stem cell therapy for cancer today. Many of those unproven cancer therapies could be considered high risk.

Available evidence suggests that CBD-rich forms of marijuana are much safer. Yet safety concerns still exist. The content of different strains and preparations is subject to many factors and in many cases is not strictly measured and controlled. The proper dose of CBD may be critical to success, but the best dose is largely unknown. The negative effects on the brain—especially in developing children—are still incompletely understood. Concerns about brain development, mood change, and memory have been expressed. Interactions with other medications including AEDs are poorly understood. The effects of stopping therapy and possible withdrawal have not been fully investigated.

This brings us to a paradox central to the current debate. Many states now allow access to medical marijuana for a wide range of medical conditions, often with limited evidence. Yet federal laws often create extraordinary barriers to obtaining the needed scientific information to support or refute this use.

Basic science studies and reports from individuals, such as Charlotte's family, about the clinical benefits of marijuana and CBD strongly support further study. A concerted effort is currently underway to make this happen. Patients and their advocates, scientists, neurologists, and major neurology societies have banded together to promote legislation to facilitate research in this area. Clinical studies of CBD compounds for epilepsy are already underway. One certainty is that more information will be available soon that may begin to remove the controversy surrounding use of marijuana and CBD.

Dietary Therapy

In the past, dietary therapy for epilepsy would have been included in the section on complementary and alternative medicine. However, it has since emerged as a more mainstream therapy. It is primarily used in the treatment of childhood epilepsy, and a few years ago would not have been included in a book about epilepsy in adolescents and adults. However, variants of diet therapy that are more suitable for adults have allowed a spread into older age groups.

Observations that fewer seizures occur in the fasting state were made centuries ago. But fasting can only be maintained for short periods of time, and this was not seen as a viable approach. It was not until about 100 years ago that a specific diet called the ketogenic diet was developed to take advantage of this observation. The ketogenic diet is a very strict diet that is high in fat and low in carbohydrates ("carbs"). Normally the processing of carbohydrates into glucose (sugar) provides fuel for the body. On a very low-carb diet, this source of energy is not available. This diet tricks the body into thinking it is in a starvation-like state. In this state, the body instead breaks down fats into compounds called ketone bodies that can also provide fuel for the body. Thus the diet is "ketogenic"—it produces ketones. The diet came into wider use in the 1990s, supported by the Charlie Foundation, an organization started by the parent of a child who benefited from the ketogenic diet. This story is powerfully told in . . . *First Do No Harm*, the 1997 movie featuring Meryl Streep.

The ketogenic diet can be very helpful and is even the treatment of choice in management of some severe childhood epilepsies. However, it is not a simple treatment. Substantial support from a dietician is needed, and the diet is usually started in the hospital to help avoid problems. Side effects on the diet can include constipation, tiredness, kidney stones, and complications from a very high fat diet, such as high cholesterol. Vitamin supplements are given to avoid vitamin deficiencies.

Use of the ketogenic diet has not spread to adolescents and adults very much. The main reason is that the extreme restrictions on carbohydrates and the high fat content make it difficult to sustain for someone used to eating a more "normal" diet. For adults who tried the diet, the dropout rate was high.

However, in the early 2000s the epilepsy group at Johns Hopkins University in Baltimore, Maryland, began publishing work on a variant of the Atkins Diet—also low carbohydrate, but less extreme—for the treatment of epilepsy. Recent studies have been encouraging, and in some cases the response to the Modified Atkins Diet (MAD) has been very similar to that of the ketogenic diet. Starting the MAD does not require hospitalization. Talk to your doctor to find out if this is a good option for you or your friend or family member. Some epilepsy centers have a dedicated dietician who helps initiate the diet and provides coaching. The book *Ketogenic Diets* by Eric Kossoff, MD, and others, is a useful resource that contains information on the MAD as well as the traditional ketogenic diet.

Chapter 13

Treatment in Special Populations and Situations

The information you have read to this point applies to most adolescents and adults with epilepsy, although it should also be clear that diagnosis and treatment must be customized to fit individual circumstances. In this chapter, we expand this customized approach to look at *groups* of people who need special consideration. The chapter opens with a review of the host of issues relevant to women with epilepsy. Next, we will review issues unique to older people with epilepsy. Then we will turn to discussing some biological and social issues that particularly affect teens with epilepsy. Finally, the last section of the chapter looks at a special *situation* in which tailored epilepsy therapy is needed: the approach to treatment of prolonged seizures, also called status epilepticus.

Women with Epilepsy

Epilepsy is about equally common in men and women. But if you are a woman with epilepsy, there are some special issues to consider. Epilepsy management in women presents potential issues throughout the lifespan and in many aspects of a woman's life.

Influence of Hormones on Seizures

During a woman's reproductive years, the menstrual cycle presents a changing pattern of hormones that can influence seizures. If a woman has a seizure pattern that is tied to hormone cycles, she is said to have **catamenial epilepsy**. Catamenial epilepsy is very common—about one-third of women show a clear relationship of the timing of seizures to the menstrual cycle.

In general, estrogen, one of the sex hormones, promotes seizure activity. Another, progesterone, is protective against seizures. During times when estrogen is high relative to progesterone, seizures may be more likely to occur. Several patterns of catamenial epilepsy have been described. The most common pattern is a higher frequency of seizures surrounding the menstrual period. Other patterns include more seizures around the time of ovulation, or in the second half of the menstrual cycle, especially if ovulation did not occur that month.

Keeping a seizure calendar can help with identifying patterns of seizures over time. Many women find it useful to chart their menstrual cycles along with seizures on a calendar. This may help with discovering whether any of the above patterns are present that could point to catamenial epilepsy.

The pattern of having more seizures around the menstrual period has been studied the most. When this pattern is seen, it can suggest some additional treatment options. With catamenial epilepsy, the seizure risk is especially elevated for certain short periods of time. This sometimes allows the use of additional focused therapy for these short time periods. This option is often more attractive than increasing the AED dose throughout the month. Intermittent use of certain AEDs to target the time around the menstrual period has been tried. Some limited support exists for use of a diuretic medication (also sometimes known as a "water pill") called acetazolamide (Diamox). Sometimes intermittent benzodiazepines, such as clobazam (Onfi) can be useful. Another approach has been to try to eliminate hormone cycles with use of hormonal therapy such as medroxyprogesterone acetate (Provera) or continuous oral contraceptives. Although potentially useful, these approaches can have their own set of side effects and potential interactions with AED therapy. Ideally, you should talk to both your neurologist and your gynecologist to decide if this is a good choice for you. Surgery (such as hysterectomy and oophorectomy) is not recommended as a treatment for catamenial epilepsy.

Finally, one other form of treatment for catamenial epilepsy—intermittent progesterone therapy—was carefully studied in a randomized controlled trial. In this study, progesterone hormone in a lozenge form was taken around the time of the menstrual period. Previous small studies had suggested that this was a very promising approach to the treatment of catamenial epilepsy. However, the study was stopped early when it became clear that progesterone therapy was not going to be clearly better than placebo. Nonetheless, those women who had a very strong catamenial pattern to their seizures (seizures more than three times more likely to occur around the menses) *did* show a response to this therapy. Thus, intermittent progesterone therapy may remain a consideration if you have a strongly catamenial epilepsy pattern.

Birth Control and AEDs

Many women with epilepsy are of childbearing age and may choose to use birth control. If you are in this group, it is very important to know about possible interactions between AEDs and some forms of birth control. Some AEDs may reduce the effectiveness of birth control. This interaction is especially important because many AEDs can also increase the risk of birth defects (see "Pregnancy and AED Therapy," this chapter).

Hormonal contraceptives are affected by some AED therapy. Hormonal contraceptives include oral contraceptives ("the pill"), as well as hormone shots or implants. As discussed in Chapter 10, some AEDs act on the liver to increase the metabolism (breakdown) of other substances. Hormones contained in birth control preparations are among those substances that can be affected by AEDs. Therefore, if you are taking an inducing AED, your hormonal birth control may be broken down more quickly and become ineffective. This can lead to breakthrough menstrual bleeding and contraceptive failure (unintended pregnancy).

AEDs that are very likely to produce this interaction are phenobarbital, primidone (Mysoline), phenytoin (Dilantin), carbamazepine (Tegretol, Tegretol XR, Carbatrol), oxcarbazepine (Trileptal and Oxtellar XR), and clobazam (Onfi), as well as high doses of topiramate (Topamax, Trokendi XR, Qudexy XR) and felbamate (Felbatol). Many of the other newer mediations do not have interactions with hormonal contraceptives and may be used together safely.

If you are taking one of these AEDs, an alternative to hormonal contraception should be considered. Some experts have suggested that using higher-dose oral contraceptives (those with at least 50 micrograms of ethinyl estradiol, common in older oral contraceptives) might still be effective, but most suggest that other forms of contraception such as an IUD or barrier methods may be more reliable.

Pregnancy and AED Therapy

Marissa is 29 years old and has well-controlled epilepsy. Her last seizure was 3 years ago when she had trouble getting her medication refilled and missed two consecutive doses of her AED (lamotrigine). She is pleased with her seizure control and lack of AED side effects. But now she and her husband are thinking about starting a family, and this has raised many

(Continued)

> (*Continued*)
> questions for her. She has heard conflicting information from family and friends. Someone told her that it is too dangerous for someone with epilepsy to go through a pregnancy. She is worried about the effects of medication on a developing baby. She wonders if she should stop her medication during the pregnancy so the baby won't be exposed. She is uncertain about whether her seizure control would worsen during pregnancy. She wonders if her children would develop seizures.

Marissa's questions and concerns are common in women with epilepsy. Many women with epilepsy are of childbearing age. The available AEDs carry an increased risk of birth defects. Most women with epilepsy cannot safely stop AED therapy during a pregnancy. Therefore it is important to know the facts, so that the best course can be charted for treatment throughout a pregnancy. The goal is to avoid problems that might be caused by AED therapy while also avoiding problems that can result from seizures during pregnancy. Management of epilepsy during pregnancy is a balancing act and requires careful attention from both an experienced obstetrician and neurologist. The good news is that the vast majority of women with epilepsy have safe pregnancies and healthy babies.

Much of our information about the safety of AEDs in pregnancy comes from pregnancy registries. These registries have been collecting information about AED use and pregnancy outcomes for years and provide the basis for much of our decision making about treatment in pregnancy (Box 13–1).

What has been learned so far? Overall, the risk of birth defects (major malformations) in children of women with epilepsy taking AEDs is about two to three times greater than in the general population. Major malformations are considered to be those that affect function or that require major intervention to correct. Common examples include cleft lip or palate, neural tube defects such as

BOX 13-1 Get Involved

The North American Antiepileptic Drug Pregnancy Registry is the main group collecting information about AEDs and pregnancy in the United States and Canada. Participation is voluntary, and you must call the toll-free number to enroll—your doctor or nurse cannot enroll you. By participating you are contributing to the effort to make future pregnancies safer for women like you who are taking AEDs.

North American AED Pregnancy Registry
www.aedpregnancyregistry.org 1-888-233-2334

Participation requires just three phone calls—once early in the pregnancy (if possible), once later, and once after delivery. Your privacy is strictly protected. Thousands of women have already participated in the registry.

spina bifida, heart defects, or abnormalities of the genital or urinary systems.

Two to three times increased risk sounds like a lot, but let's look at the numbers. For healthy women who don't have epilepsy and who are not taking AEDs, the risk of these major malformations is about 1 to 3 percent. For women with epilepsy taking AEDs, it is roughly 3 to 9 percent. Thus even though the risk is two to three times greater, the vast majority of pregnancies in women with epilepsy (more than 90 percent) are free of major malformations.

What can be done to minimize the risk?

- Take a folic acid supplement. Folic acid is a vitamin supplement that is recommended for all pregnant women. It may be especially important for women taking AEDs, some of which may deplete folic acid. Because having adequate folic acid is important very early in the pregnancy, it is recommended that all women with epilepsy of childbearing age take a folic acid supplement at all times as a general health measure. The dose has not been scientifically determined, but most authorities suggest that women with epilepsy take at least 1 mg per day and that women taking higher-risk AEDs such as valproate take up to 5 mg per day. Talk to your doctor about what is right for you.

- If possible, avoid AEDs that have a particularly high risk of birth defects. The worst of these appears to be valproate, which most people take as sodium valproate (Depakote), but sometimes as valproic acid (Depakene). Several pregnancy registries have identified this as the AED most likely to produce birth defects. The North American AED Pregnancy Registry has also released information identifying phenobarbital and topiramate (Topamax) as higher-risk medications.

- Use single-drug therapy (monotherapy) rather than multiple AED therapy (polytherapy) whenever possible, as some combinations of AEDs create increased risk of birth defects.

- If you have been seizure free for many years, talk with your doctor about whether it is safe to consider tapering off of your AED. If this is a consideration, it should be done in advance of a planned pregnancy.

- Do not stop your AED during pregnancy out of fear that the AED might be causing harm to the developing baby. This could result in worsening seizures, which could be harmful to both you and the baby.

Recent studies have looked beyond major malformations to more subtle issues of the effects of AEDs on brain development. Much of what has been learned is reassuring, but exposure to one specific drug during pregnancy (sodium valproate [Depakote]) is associated with lower IQ in exposed infants, even when tested at age 6, many years after the exposure. It is one more reason why sodium valproate (Depakote) should be avoided if at all possible during pregnancy.

Seizure control can be variable during pregnancy. Being seizure free in the year before pregnancy is a good predictor of being seizure free during pregnancy. Seizure frequency in pregnancy remains unchanged for most women. It may improve in a minority and can worsen in anywhere from a one-fifth to one-third of women.

Some of the changes in seizure frequency during pregnancy can be attributed to changes in AED levels. Several physical changes during pregnancy can affect the levels of certain AEDs. The most dramatic changes can be seen with lamotrigine. Changes in the metabolism of lamotrigine during pregnancy can produce marked decreases in lamotrigine levels, and large increases in dose may be needed just to maintain the usual blood level and degree of seizure protection. If you are taking lamotrigine, your doctor will probably want to monitor your AED levels closely throughout your pregnancy. If changes were made in dosing, these changes will likely need to be carefully reversed following delivery.

What does all of this mean for Marissa?

Marissa scheduled a clinic visit with her neurologist. Her husband came with her, and they devoted the entire meeting to discussing pregnancy planning. Marissa left the meeting feeling more informed and less worried. She learned that most women with epilepsy have successful, healthy pregnancies. She reviewed the information from pregnancy registries and found that her AED (lamotrigine) appeared to be one of the safer AEDs in pregnancy. She was already taking a folate vitamin supplement and understood the importance

(*Continued*)

(*Continued*)

of continuing it. She and her doctor decided it was safest to not stop her seizure medication during pregnancy, because in the past she had had a seizure when she missed just two doses. She was reassured that her good seizure control predicted continued good seizure control throughout a pregnancy. She understood that her lamotrigine levels would need to be checked frequently throughout a pregnancy, that dose increases would likely be needed to maintain the same AED levels, and that dose reductions would then be needed following delivery.

Marissa's story is just one story that shows how information about pregnancy in women with epilepsy can be useful. If you are on different AED therapy, have poorly controlled seizures, or other individual differences, your planning for pregnancy might look different. But the important principle is that getting the facts and talking them over can address some of your worries and make things as safe as possible for you and your baby.

Information about AEDs and pregnancy changes frequently. A good resource for current updates is the website of the North American AED Pregnancy Registry at www.aedpregnancyregistry.org.

Reproductive Function

We have seen in Chapter 10 that some AED therapy can result in sexual dysfunction in both men and women. Women with epilepsy also have lower than expected fertility rates (lower chances of successfully having children). Studies show mixed findings regarding the cause of reduced fertility. Seizures themselves may disrupt the normal patterns of release of sex hormones. This can cause problems with ovulation and normal reproductive function. AEDs may also contribute to decreased fertility in women with epilepsy. If this is an issue for you, an evaluation for common causes of infertility as well as causes related to your epilepsy and medications should be undertaken.

Menopause

Changes in seizure patterns can be seen near the end of the reproductive years. Perimenopause, the transition to menopause, is marked by fluctuations in hormones and is sometimes associated with increased seizures. During menopause, when hormones are more stable, seizures may improve, especially in women who previously had a catamenial pattern of seizures. There is good evidence that hormone replacement can increase seizures. If you are considering hormone replacement therapy, it is a good idea to include your neurologist in the discussion.

Bone Health

Bone health is really an issue for both men and women with epilepsy, but because women are more prone to problems with bone health, it is often considered a women's health issue.

Two terms are important to know. **Osteopenia** refers to bone density that is below average but not severe enough to be called osteoporosis. **Osteoporosis** is a more marked thinning of the bones that clearly increases the person's risk of fractures (broken bones).

What does this have to do with epilepsy and AEDs? The risk of fractures is clearly elevated in people with epilepsy. Some of this risk is related to greater odds of falling, because of seizures. But several AEDs can also accelerate the process of bone thinning so that osteoporosis may be seen at ages much younger than expected. Most of the problem appears to be related to the enzyme-inducing AEDs (EIAEDs) mentioned in Chapter 10. These are AEDs that cause the liver to break down other medications more quickly, including hormones and some vitamins. The strongest EIAEDs are older drugs such as phenobarbital, phenytoin (Dilantin), and carbamazepine (Tegretol). They may accelerate bone loss in several ways. One important way is by breaking down vitamin D more rapidly. Vitamin D is important for maintaining bone heath, and low vitamin D levels can lead to poor bone health. But faster breakdown of vitamin D is not the whole story. A pattern of earlier bone loss has also been noted with valproate (Depakote), which is not an EIAED. Scientists are continuing to work to understand how AEDs affect bone health so that countermeasures can be put into place and problems avoided.

If you have been on an AED, especially an EIAED, for more than 5 years, your doctor might want to consider performing a test of bone density called a dual-energy X-ray absorptiometry (DXA) scan, regardless of your age. Depending on your situation, supplements of vitamin D and calcium or even a change of AED therapy might be considered if abnormalities are found.

Older People with Epilepsy

Virginia is 68 years old. Over the years she had experienced her share of health issues—high blood pressure, diabetes, breathing problems from many years of smoking, and, last year, a stroke that made her left arm and leg weak. But she had recovered pretty well, and was back home, getting around fine, and just using a cane if she needed to walk longer distances. Her thinking was still very sharp. However, several months after her stroke she began having episodes of confusion that lasted a few minutes. Her son was with her when the third one happened. He observed that she was fine one minute and then

(Continued)

(Continued)

abruptly became confused and unresponsive. She did not fall or pass out. After several minutes she became more responsive but had no memory of what had happened, and she felt tired and a little "fuzzy" with her thinking the rest of the day. Virginia saw her primary care doctor and then a neurologist, who recognized that these were seizures that resulted from the brain injury she had sustained when she had her stroke. Her neurologist gave her a diagnosis of epilepsy.

Virginia did not expect that she would have her first seizure at age 68, and even though her neurologist told her that she had epilepsy, she didn't really believe it. She thought: *Isn't epilepsy something that children get?*

As noted, people over age 65 make up the largest group of people with epilepsy, outnumbering even children with epilepsy. This pattern is not likely to change; our aging population means there will be greater numbers of older people with epilepsy.

Epilepsy may be a more challenging diagnosis to make in the elderly. Sometimes doctors are slow to consider the diagnosis, as competing problems like heart rhythm disturbances and transient ischemic attacks (TIAs, or "mini-strokes") are common in this age group. The seizures themselves may be more subtle in older people, with simple staring spells lacking well-defined auras and automatisms.

Once a diagnosis of epilepsy is established, the goals of treatment are the same as for anyone with epilepsy: to be seizure free with no side effects. However, there are many treatment principles that are especially important in an older population:

- When starting AEDs it is necessary to "start low and go slow." Older people may not metabolize medications as quickly, and changes in kidney function can affect that rate at which some AEDs are cleared from the body.

- It is important to avoid AEDs that are prone to drug–drug interactions. Some studies have found that the elderly take an average of 8 to 13 prescription medications. Adding an AED with multiple drug interactions to that mix is asking for trouble.
- Consider other health issues. These may have a lot of influence on AED prescribing:
  - Osteoporosis (avoid older and enzyme-inducing AEDs)
  - Decreased kidney function (reduce doses of those AEDs cleared by the kidneys)
  - Cognitive (thinking) problems or dementia (avoid AEDs likely to worsen memory and thinking)
  - Falls (if at risk for falls, avoid AEDs likely to cause dizziness or balance problems)
- Depression or mood issues (avoid AEDs likely to worsen mood or depression)
- Tolerability is important. Older people tend to be more sensitive to the side effects of AEDs.

This last point was emphasized by a study of AED treatment in older veterans with a new diagnosis of epilepsy, reported in 2005. It compared a standard older AED (carbamazepine [Tegretol]) to two newer AEDs (gabapentin [Neurontin] and lamotrigine [Lamictal]). All provided similar seizure control. However, gabapentin (Neurontin) and lamotrigine (Lamictal) were better tolerated and thus resulted in more successful treatment. Similar findings have been seen in studies of other of the newer AEDs, including levetiracetam (Keppra).

Let's revisit Virginia's situation.

Virginia's primary care doctor started her on phenytoin (Dilantin), a medication that he was familiar with. It didn't take long to find out that she felt terrible. She was tired,

(Continued)

(*Continued*)

dizzy, and her blood thinner medication was no longer working because of medication interactions, and the dose had to be doubled. There were also interactions with her cholesterol medicine. She saw a neurologist, who listened to her concerns and converted her to treatment with lamotrigine. At relatively low doses she is feeling well and is seizure free.

Teens with Epilepsy

Epilepsy in the teenage years is common. Despite this, surprisingly little research has been conducted specific to management of epilepsy in the teenage years. The teen years seem to exist in a borderland zone—some studies of children include teens, while many studies of epilepsy in adults may also include teens. Physical and psychological development also spans these groups and may overlap with both children and adults. Older teens may be physically and physiologically very similar to adults. Many teens have also developed a level of psychological maturity similar to young adults. But there is a large range, and especially early teens may share more physical and psychological characteristics with older children. If you are an adult, you probably remember that the inevitable changes through teen years present substantial psychological and social challenges. These are magnified if the challenges of having epilepsy also have to be navigated.

The hormonal changes of the preteen and teenage years can have a profound influence on seizures. Some epilepsy syndromes, such as juvenile absence epilepsy and juvenile myoclonic epilepsy, may first appear during early teenage years. Focal epilepsies can appear, and some refractory focal epilepsies, previously better controlled in childhood, can become difficult to manage beginning in the early teens.

The opposite effect can also be seen: Adolescence may signal the end of active epilepsy in some other epilepsy syndromes. Certain syndromes such as childhood absence epilepsy and **benign epilepsy with centrotemporal spikes** may reliably become inactive during adolescence and beyond.

During the teenage years, brain development is also continuing. Much of what is thought of by adults as "teenage behavior" is directly tied to these continuing changes in the brain. Teens are not simply younger or smaller adults. Ongoing changes, especially in the frontal lobes of the brain, may explain differences in judgment, risk taking, and the ability to control impulses.

At times, the social and behavioral issues of the teenage years can affect treatment. As in adults, the most common approach to therapy is with AEDs, but maintaining regular dosing of AEDs can be challenging in teens. This can be a time of separating oneself as an individual, and "battles of will" can be set up between parents who "nag" their teens to take their AEDs, and teens who may at times appear less concerned about the importance of regular dosing. Good and open lines of communication between the teen and doctor are critical. It is important to explain carefully the reasons why treatment is needed, why a particular medication was chosen, why regular dosing is important, and to be open to discussions of alternatives when appropriate. In my experience, most teens will greatly appreciate having these "adult" discussions with their doctor. Opportunities for discussion with the teen when the parents are outside of the exam room may also be helpful, as these are times when important questions about substance use, birth control, and sexuality may come up. Those issues can directly affect choice of therapy for epilepsy, seizure control, and contraceptive choices.

If possible, selection of an AED that requires relatively infrequent dosing may be advantageous. As with adults, we try to minimize side effects of AEDs. In teens, learning and mood are especially critical issues. All efforts should be made to choose an AED that will not impair thinking and learning. Some research has shown that mood disturbances and suicidality are common in teens. Changes in behavior should not be simply attributed to teenage "moodiness" and should be addressed promptly. Mood, as much as seizure control, is directly tied to quality of life in teens (and everyone) with epilepsy.

Treatment in Special Situations: Status Epilepticus

In Chapter 2 I introduced the idea that, although rare, seizures can be prolonged, lasting 30 minutes or more. In addition, repeated seizures without recovery between events can occur and may last for 30 minutes or more. Both of these circumstances are termed status epilepticus, and this is almost always considered a medical emergency.

Much of the treatment of status epilepticus is done in the hospital or intensive care unit (ICU) setting. Many different medications can be used to treat status epilepticus. These include intravenous (IV) forms of several common AEDs, as well as other medications that are more commonly used as anesthesia. If you or someone you know has been diagnosed with status epilepticus, your doctor will want to rapidly get control of the seizures to prevent injury to body systems and the brain that can occur with prolonged seizures. Discussion of these hospital-based treatment approaches for prolonged seizures is beyond the scope of this book. However, there are some important things for you to know and some actions that you can take to reduce the risk of status epilepticus.

As discussed in Chapter 2, some instances of status epilepticus in people with preexisting epilepsy are triggered by missed doses of AEDs or abrupt stopping of AED therapy. Thus, the first principle of status epilepticus prevention is to avoid these situations that increase the risk of status. Anyone who has tried taking daily medicine for weeks, let alone years, will know that it is very difficult to be perfect and never miss a dose of medication. We are all human, and occasional missed or late doses can happen. But the less this happens, the lower the chances of status epilepticus.

If you have had repetitive or prolonged seizures in the past or are felt to be especially prone to these problems, there are some AED approaches that can help prevent status epilepticus and reduce the need for emergency treatment. Your doctor may consider prescribing a benzodiazepine medication such as lorazepam (Ativan) that you can take by mouth if you start having a cluster of seizures. This requires you to be awake enough to safely take medication by mouth and is not a good approach for true status epilepticus. However, when swallowed or dissolved under the tongue, these medications can provide several hours of additional protection against further seizures, but it may take 30 minutes or more to take effect and 2 hours to reach peak effect.

For more urgent treatment, especially for prolonged or clustered seizures when a person is not awake enough to safely take a medication by mouth, another way of dosing medication can be used. Medication given by rectal dosing can be rapidly absorbed. There is a rectal form of diazepam (Valium) with the brand name of Diastat. It is prescribed in preloaded syringes in a gel form. The syringe has a soft tip. A family member or caregiver can be instructed on how to insert the soft-tipped syringe and deliver a fixed dose of diazepam rectally.

This form of therapy has been more widely adopted and successfully used in children. In an adult having seizures, rectal administration of medication can be more challenging. In many settings (for example, in a restaurant or other public place), rectal administration may be difficult or impossible. For these reasons, other forms of rapidly absorbed medications for use in acute seizures are being developed. These include medications that can be dosed using a nasal spray. Other forms can be given at home as a preloaded shot in a large muscle using an auto-injector, much like the "EpiPen" that is used when someone has a sudden allergic reaction. If intranasal and intramuscular dosing of acute therapy for seizures are approved, they would be welcome additional to the toolkit available to treat acute seizures.

None of these measures replaces emergency care. Whether or not acute therapy has been given, continued seizures or continued decreased or lack of responsiveness is still a reason to call 911 and get emergency help (see also seizure first aid in Chapter 3).

Absence seizure: A generalized seizure type usually seen in children characterized by a brief loss of awareness, usually for seconds, with rapid return to normal.

Action potential: The name given to the firing or output of a brain cell (neuron).

AED: See *antiepileptic drug.*

Ambulatory electroencephalogram (EEG): A long-term (often 24 hour) EEG study performed in the home environment. The EEG recording is typically started at the hospital or clinic, and the patient returns the next day to remove the recording equipment and have the EEG interpreted.

Angiogram: A method of imaging blood vessels accomplished by injecting dye into a blood vessel and using X-rays to create pictures of the arteries and veins.

Anterior temporal lobectomy (ATL): A form of epilepsy surgery in which the anterior (front) and middle portions of the temporal lobe are surgically removed in order to remove the seizure focus and stop seizures.

Antiepileptic drug (AED): A medication used to prevent or reduce the frequency of epileptic seizures.

Arteriovenous malformation (AVM): An abnormal connection between arteries and veins that poses a risk of bleeding and that can be a cause of epilepsy.

ATL: See *anterior temporal lobectomy*.

Automatism: An automatic behavior that occurs during a seizure, often during a complex partial seizure.

AVM: See *arteriovenous malformation*.

Benign epilepsy with centrotemporal spikes: A common epilepsy syndrome that usually begins in childhood and resolves in adolescence or early adulthood.

Brain mapping: A form of testing that assigns specific functions to specific regions of the brain in order to identify areas that should be spared during an epilepsy surgery.

Brainstem: The lower part of the brain, which is responsible for controlling automatic functions such as breathing and heart rate, among other functions.

Broad-spectrum antiepileptic drug (AED): An AED that is effective in treating both focal-onset and generalized-from-onset seizures.

CAM: See *complementary and alternative medicine*.

CAT scan: See *computed tomography*.

CBD: See *cannabidiol*.

Cannabidiol (CBD): The main non-psychoactive component of marijuana that is being investigated for antiepileptic properties.

Catamenial epilepsy: A pattern of seizures in women that is closely tied to hormonal changes of the menstrual cycle.

Cavernous hemangioma: A blood vessel malformation containing a collection of thin-walled veins that is prone to bleeding and that can be a cause of epilepsy.

Complementary and alternative medicine (CAM): Medical therapy that is outside the realm of traditional medicine. Complementary medicine is used together with traditional medicine, and alternative medicine is used in place of it.

Complex partial seizure: A focal seizure that causes confusion or impairment of consciousness.

Computed tomography: A method of imaging the brain using X-ray technology. Also known as a *CT* or *CAT scan*.

Concordant: A term used to describe tests in an epilepsy surgery evaluation that are in agreement and consistently point to the same area as representing the seizure focus.

Conversion disorder: A psychiatric condition in which psychological and emotional stresses or traumas are converted (unconsciously) into physical symptoms, including seizure-like events.

Convulsive syncope: An episode of syncope (see *syncope*) in which blood flow to the brain is not promptly restored, and the syncope is accompanied by body stiffening or jerking movements.

Corpus callosotomy: A form of epilepsy surgery that involves cutting part or most of the connections between the two halves (hemispheres) of the brain.

Corpus callosum: The thick bundle of nerve fibers that is the main connection between the two halves (hemispheres) of the brain.

Cortex: The outer, wrinkled surface of the brain that contains most of the nerve cells (neurons) in the brain. Most seizures originate in the cortex.

Cortical stimulation mapping: A method of identifying areas of important brain function by delivering small amounts of electrical stimulation while having the patient perform a task. This type of brain mapping is often performed as part of intracranial EEG monitoring.

CT scan: See *computed tomography*.

DBS: See *deep brain stimulation*.

Deep brain stimulation (DBS): A method of electrical stimulation to a deep brain focus to treat a medical condition such as Parkinson's disease or epilepsy.

Depth electrodes: Long, thin EEG electrodes that are specially designed to record from deep areas of the brain.

Differential diagnosis: The range of diagnoses being considered in a person with a given set of symptoms before the list is narrowed and a specific diagnosis is made.

Diffusion tensor imaging (DTI): An MRI technique to map the white matter pathways (the "wiring") of the brain.

Drop seizure: A type of seizure that causes a sudden fall, usually the result of a tonic or atonic seizure.

DTI: See *diffusion tensor imaging.*

EEG: See *electroencephalogram.*

EIAED: See *enzyme-inducing antiepileptic drugs.*

Electroencephalogram: A test of electrical brain wave activity.

Enzyme-inducing antiepileptic drugs (EIAEDs): Those AEDs that act on the liver to increase the metabolism of other substances, such as other medications (for example, birth control pills, blood thinners) or other substances in the body (for example, hormones, vitamins).

Epilepsy: A condition of recurring, unprovoked seizures. The diagnosis is usually made after someone has had more than one unprovoked seizure. Epilepsy can also be diagnosed after a single seizure in someone who is at high risk of having more seizures.

Epilepsy syndrome: A group of features that usually occur together and characterize a particular condition. An epilepsy syndrome takes into account seizure types, but also information from the patient's history, examination, and test results.

Epileptiform discharge: Sometimes called a "spike" or a "sharp wave," this is a finding often seen on the EEG of someone who has epilepsy. The epileptiform discharge does not cause symptoms (it lasts for just a fraction of a second) but is a marker for epilepsy and may help to define the seizure type and epilepsy syndrome.

Excitatory neurotransmitter: A neurotransmitter is a brain chemical that helps transmit a signal in the brain. An excitatory neurotransmitter is one that sends a signal for other connected brain cells to fire.

Executive function: The aspects of brain function that involve planning, problem solving, and higher-level decision making.

Extratemporal epilepsy: A form of focal epilepsy in which seizures begin in a focus outside of the temporal lobe.

Febrile seizure: A seizure type that is considered to be a provoked seizure—provoked by high body temperature. Febrile seizures usually occur between the ages of 6 months and 5 years.

fMRI: See *functional MRI*.

Focal cortical dysplasia: An area of abnormality in a focal part of the brain that is the result of abnormal brain development in that area. This is a common cause of seizures.

Focal seizure (see also *partial seizure*): A seizure that begins in a particular brain region, in contrast to a generalized-from-onset seizure.

Functional MRI (fMRI): A specialized type of MRI scan that displays brain areas that are activated during a particular task, such as identification of motor areas of the brain activated by finger tapping.

GABA (gamma-aminobutyric acid): The main inhibitory neurotransmitter in the brain.

Generalized seizure: A group of seizure types that seem to begin in the whole brain at once, in contrast to *partial* or *focal seizures* that begin in a particular place or region of the brain.

Generalized tonic-clonic (GTC) seizure: A severe seizure type that includes a phase of body stiffening (tonic) and jerking (clonic). A GTC seizure can result from spread of a focal-onset seizure or can be generalized from onset. Previously called a *grand mal seizure*.

Glutamate: The main excitatory neurotransmitter in the brain.

Grand mal seizure: Old term for what is now called a *generalized tonic-clonic (GTC) seizure*.

Gray matter: The parts of the brain that contain nerve cells (*neurons*), in contrast to *white matter*, which contains the connections or "wiring" between neurons.

Grid electrodes: An array of EEG recording electrodes embedded in a thin, flexible plastic sheet that can be placed by a surgeon to record EEG signals directly from the surface of the brain.

GTC: See *generalized tonic clonic seizure.*

Hemisphere: One half of the brain.

Hemorrhagic stroke: A type of stroke that involves bleeding into or around the brain.

Hippocampus: Part of the medial (deep) portion of the temporal lobe. This part of the brain has a specialized function that is important for short-term memory and is a part of the brain that is commonly involved in seizure onset.

Hypersynchronous: A condition in which the firing of brain cells is excessively synchronized, as in an epileptic seizure.

Hysterical seizure: An old term for a *psychogenic nonepileptic seizure (PNES)* that should be abandoned.

IAP: See *intracarotid amobarbital procedure, Wada test.*

Ictal: A medical term that refers to a seizure, in contrast to *interictal,* which means between seizures.

Inducer: A medication that speeds up the metabolism (breakdown) or clearance of other medications or substances in the body.

Inhibitor: A medication that slows down the metabolism (breakdown) or clearance of other medications or substances in the body.

Inhibitory neurotransmitter: A neurotransmitter is a brain chemical that helps transmit a signal in the brain. An inhibitory neurotransmitter is one that inhibits or prevents other connected brain cells from firing.

Interictal: In between seizures.

Intracarotid amobarbital procedure (IAP): See *Wada test.*

Intracranial EEG: Specialized EEG testing that is accomplished by placing recording electrodes directly in or on the surface of the brain.

Ischemic stroke: A type of stroke that results from lack of blood flow to a part of the brain.

Juvenile myoclonic epilepsy (JME): An epilepsy syndrome that often begins in adolescence and that is characterized by myoclonic, generalized tonic-clonic, and sometimes absence seizures.

JME: See *juvenile myoclonic epilepsy.*

Lennox-Gastaut syndrome: An epilepsy syndrome in the category of symptomatic generalized epilepsies. People with this epilepsy syndrome often have some degree of intellectual disability, a certain pattern on their EEG called slow spike-and-wave, and often several types of generalized-from-onset seizures, although all of these features are not needed to establish the syndrome diagnosis.

LGS: See *Lennox-Gastaut syndrome.*

Magnetic resonance imaging (MRI): An imaging method that uses a strong magnet to produce detailed pictures of the brain.

Magnetoencephalography (MEG): A test that uses similar principles as the electroencephalogram (EEG), but instead of measuring the electrical activity of the brain, it measures the corresponding magnetic activity.

Medically refractory epilepsy (see also medication-resistant epilepsy): Any epilepsy that is resistant to treatment with AEDs and where seizures continue despite medical treatment. People with medically refractory epilepsy are often considered for epilepsy surgery, medical devices, or other alternative treatments when AED therapy fails.

Medication-resistant epilepsy (see also medically refractory epilepsy): Any epilepsy that is resistant to treatment with AEDs and where seizures continue despite medical treatment. People with medically refractory epilepsy are often considered for epilepsy surgery, medical devices, or other alternative treatments when AED therapy fails.

MEG: See *magnetoencephalography.*

Mesial temporal sclerosis: A form of injury to the mesial (medial, or middle) portion of the temporal lobe that results in loss of neurons in that area and an increase in the numbers of other support cells (glia), resulting in a "scar." The rewiring of this brain region in response to this injury commonly produces seizures that can be difficult to control with AEDs.

Metastatic tumor: A tumor that spreads from its initial source, such as a lung tumor that spreads to the brain.

Monotherapy: Treatment with a single AED.

MRI: See *magnetic resonance imaging.*

MTS: See *mesial temporal sclerosis.*

Mutation: A change in a gene that can lead to disease, including epilepsy.

Narrow-spectrum AED: An antiepileptic medication that works specifically to treat focal but not generalized epilepsy.

Network: A highly interconnected group of neurons (brain cells).

Neuron: A cell that is specialized for sending signals as part of the nervous system; a "brain cell."

Neuropsychologist: A medical professional who specializes in assessing and treating cognitive and psychological problems.

Neurotransmitter: A chemical messenger in the brain that carries a signal from one brain cell (neuron) to another brain cell with which it is connected.

Off-label: The use of a medication for purposes other than those officially approved by the US Food and Drug Administration (FDA).

Osteopenia: A mild reduction in bone density (thinning of the bones) that is below average for age but not severe enough to constitute osteoporosis (see *osteoporosis*).

Osteoporosis: A significant reduction in bone density that places people at higher risk for fractures. Long-term use of several AEDs can be risk factors for developing osteoporosis.

Partial seizure (see also *focal seizure*): A seizure that begins in a particular brain region, in contrast to a generalized-from-onset seizure.

PET: See *positron emission tomography.*

Pharmacogenomics: The science of the genetics of responses to medications.

Polytherapy: Treatment with more than one AED simultaneously.

Positron emission tomography (PET): A specialized imaging test that produces pictures of the brain based on metabolic activity. It images the function rather than the structure of the brain.

Postictal psychosis: Symptoms of psychosis that emerge following a seizure or cluster of seizures, and then go away for long periods of time between seizures.

Postictal state: The period immediately following a seizure when the brain is recovering from the seizure. This time period is often marked by confusion.

Primary brain tumor: A brain tumor that arises directly from brain cells (as opposed to a brain tumor that results from spread of tumor from another location, such as spread of lung cancer).

Provoked seizure: A seizure triggered by some strong external stimulus in a person who does not necessarily have an ongoing tendency to have seizures.

Pseudoseizure: An old term for a *psychogenic nonepileptic seizure (PNES)* that should be abandoned.

Psychogenic nonepileptic seizure (PNES): A seizure-like event that is behavioral rather than epileptic in origin. A psychogenic nonepileptic seizure is not associated with an abnormal brain discharges and needs to be treated differently from an epileptic seizure.

Radiologist: A medical doctor who specializes in interpreting imaging studies. A neuro-radiologist specializes in imaging studies of the brain and spine.

Randomized controlled trial (RCT): A study method in which participants are randomly assigned (as with a coin toss) to either an active treatment or a treatment that is not expected to help, called a placebo. If those in the active treatment group do better than the placebo group, there is convincing evidence that the therapy works.

Responsive neurostimulation (RNS): A method of treating epilepsy by delivering electrical stimulation of the seizure focus when onset of a seizure is detected.

RCT: See *randomized controlled trial.*

REM behavior disorder: A sleep disorder in which the individual "acts out his dreams," often with violent, thrashing behaviors.

RNS: See *responsive neurostimulation.*

SAH: See *selective amygdalohippocampectomy.*

Secondarily generalized tonic-clonic seizure: A seizure that begins as a focal seizure but then spreads to involve the whole brain and leads to stiffening and then convulsive or jerking movements of the body.

Seizure: Paroxysmal uncontrolled electrical activity in the brain causing a variety of symptoms depending on the seizure type, area of onset, and pattern of spread.

Selective amygdalohippocampectomy (SAH): An epilepsy surgery technique that represents an alternative to anterior temporal lobectomy. With SAH, the medial temporal lobe structures are targeted for selective removal, and the remainder of the temporal lobe is unaffected.

Signs: Features that can be identified by an external observer (in contrast to *symptoms,* which are what the patient experiences).

Sharp wave: An abnormal finding on EEG that indicates an increased risk of seizures.

Simple partial seizure: A focal seizure in which consciousness is preserved.

Single-photon emission computed tomography (SPECT): A nuclear medicine imaging study that takes pictures of the brain based on the amount of blood flow to various regions of the brain. If performed between seizures (interictal SPECT), this may show decreased blood flow in the area of the seizure focus. If performed during a seizure (ictal SPECT), this may show increased blood flow at the seizure focus.

SISCOM: See *subtraction ictal SPECT coregistered to MRI.*

SPECT: See *single-photon emission computed tomography.*

Spike: An abnormal finding on EEG that indicates an increased risk of seizures.

Spinal cord: A part of the central nervous system. The spinal cord is a cylinder-shaped bundle of neurons and nerve fibers that provides a connection between the body and the brain.

Status epilepticus: A condition marked by prolonged seizures, usually defined as a single seizure lasting more than 30 minutes or a series of seizures without recovery between seizures lasting 30 minutes or longer. This is generally considered a medical emergency requiring emergency treatment to stop seizures.

Stereotactic radiosurgery: A form of "surgical" treatment that uses focused radiation beams to treat abnormal tissue. This technique avoids the need for a surgical incision and open surgery.

Stevens-Johnson syndrome: A serious, potentially life-threatening allergic reaction to a drug.

Strip electrodes: Specialized EEG recording electrodes that can be placed directly on the surface of the brain by a surgeon to accomplish intracranial recording.

Subtraction ictal SPECT coregistered to MRI (SISCOM): A nuclear medicine imaging tool that is used to help locate a seizure focus prior to epilepsy surgery. It consists of matching and subtracting two SPECT scan images—one performed during a seizure (ictal SPECT) and one performed between seizures (interictal SPECT). The result of the subtraction (the seizure focus) is overlaid on an MRI scan so the location in the brain can be easily identified. See also SPECT.

Sudden unexpected death in epilepsy (SUDEP): A term that refers to the higher than expected risk of sudden death in people with epilepsy. This condition is discussed in detail in Chapter 3.

SUDEP: See *sudden unexpected death in epilepsy*.

Symptoms: Changes in the mind or body that a patient experiences (in contrast to *signs*, which are what an external person observes).

Synapse: The point of connection between neurons (brain cells) that allows transmission of signals and communication.

Syncope: A fainting episode that could be mistaken for a seizure.

THC: The main psychoactive component of marijuana (the component most responsible for the "high").

TIA: See *transient ischemic attack.*

Todd's paralysis: Temporary weakness of a limb or one side of the body following a seizure. The side of the body opposite the seizure onset in the brain is most often affected.

Toxic epidermal necrolysis: A serious, potentially life-threatening allergic reaction to a drug.

Transient ischemic attack (TIA): A "mini-stroke" or stroke-like symptoms caused by blockage of blood flow to part of the brain that reverses before permanent brain injury occurs.

Traumatic brain injury: An injury to the brain as a result of trauma that may lead to development of epilepsy. The most common causes of traumatic brain injury that lead to seizures are motor vehicle accidents, violence, and falls.

Vagus nerve stimulation (VNS): A surgically implanted medical device that treats seizures by delivering intermittent pulses of electrical stimulation to one of the cranial nerves in the neck called the vagus nerve.

Video-EEG monitoring: A diagnostic test that includes a prolonged EEG recording with simultaneous recording of video. The goal is usually to record seizures and document both the visual appearance of the seizure and the associated brain wave changes.

VNS: See *vagus nerve stimulation.*

Wada test: A test that is sometimes part of the epilepsy presurgical evaluation, in which one-half of the brain is briefly "put to sleep," while language and memory tests are administered. The test helps to locate which half of the brain is most important for language function and can provide important information about memory function. (Also called *intracarotid amobarbital procedure.*)

White matter: The "wiring" or "cables" that connect neurons (brain cells) in different brain regions.

Other Reading and Resources

General Epilepsy

Bromfield EB, Cavazos JE, Sirven JI, eds. Basic mechanisms underlying seizures and epilepsy. In: *An Introduction to Epilepsy* [Internet]. West Hartford, CT: American Epilepsy Society, 2006. Available from: http://www.ncbi.nlm.nih.gov/books/NBK2510/

Scharfman, H. The neurobiology of epilepsy. *Curr Neurol Neurosci Rep.* 2007;7(4):348–354. http://www.ncbi.nlm.nih.gov/pmc/articles/PMC2492886/

Epilepsy Surgery

If you or someone you know would like to know more about epilepsy surgery or locate a surgical epilepsy center near you, the best resource is the website of the National Association of Epilepsy Centers (NAEC; www.naec-epilepsy.org). These centers are also excellent resources for expert medical care of epilepsy.

Complementary and Alternative Medicine (CAM) in Epilepsy

Devinsky O, Schachter SC, Pacia SV. *Alternative Therapies for Epilepsy Care*. New York: Demos Medical Publishing; 2012.

National Center for Complementary and Integrative Health website. http://nccam.nih.gov/.

Psychogenic Nonepileptic Seizures (PNES)

There are some excellent sources of additional information on psychogenic nonepileptic seizures (PNES):

Epilepsy Foundation: Types of Seizures. Updated November 2013. http://www.epilepsy.com/learn/types-seizures/non-epilepsy-seizures.

Benbadis SR, Heriaud L. *Psychogenic (Non-Epileptic) Seizures: A Guide for Patients & Families*. Tampa, FL: University of South Florida; date unknown. http://hsc.usf.edu/com/epilepsy/PNESbrochure.pdf.

Seizure First Aid

Epilepsy Foundation: http://www.epilepsy.com/firstaid

Driving and Epilepsy

Epilepsy Foundation: www.epilepsy.com/driving-laws

Employment Issues

Epilepsy Foundation: http://www.epilepsy.com/get-help/managing-your-epilepsy/independent-living/employment

Information about Sudden Unexpected Death in Epilepsy (SUDEP)

Partners Against Mortality in Epilepsy: pame.aesnet.org

Electronic Seizure Diary

"My Epilepsy Diary" at www.epilepsy.com.

APPENDIX 2

Information about Specific Antiepileptic Drugs

As noted in Chapter 5, additional information about specific anti-epileptic drugs (AEDs) can be found here. The reason for including this information here is to avoid distracting from the discussion of general principles of AED choice, management, interactions, and side effects. With too many details, the forest can be lost for the trees. This appendix is *not* intended to be an exhaustive list of every fact about every AED. That would require another book! It would also be quickly out of date, as information about medications is constantly changing and being updated. Instead, some selected common or important features of each drug are mentioned.

This appendix is meant as a starting point to encourage discussions with your doctor. Please also keep in mind that information about medications can change as new data become available, so please check with your doctor, pharmacist, or the manufacturer of the medication for the most up-to-date information. Another good resource for more complete reference information about medications is at epilepsy.com.

Carbamazepine (Tegretol), Carbamazepine Extended Release (Carbatrol, Tegretol XR)

This medication is used for the treatment of focal-onset (including secondarily generalized tonic-clonic) seizures. It can potentially worsen seizures in people with generalized-from-onset seizure types.

The regular form of carbamazepine should be given three times daily; extended release forms have the advantage of twice daily dosing. It is metabolized by the liver and is an enzyme-inducing AED (EIAED), which means it can have interactions with many other medications (both AEDs and non-AEDs). It must be started at a low dose because the body breaks it down slowly at first, then speeds up breakdown after a couple of weeks.

Common doses are in the range of 600 mg to 1200 mg per day, and blood levels of about 4 to 12 mcg/mL are often targeted. Dose-related side effects (if the dose is too high) can commonly include double vision, dizziness, drowsiness, trouble with balance, or nausea. Treatment with carbamazepine may result in low blood sodium levels. It can cause decreases in blood counts or severe rashes.

Clobazam (Onfi)

This medication is approved for use for seizures related to Lennox-Gastaut syndrome in people over age 2. It is used "off label" at times for other seizure types.

A dose of clobazam stays in the body for a long time (long "half-life"). It is usually dosed twice daily, often starting at a low dose (around 5 mg) and increasing to a usual maximum of 40 mg per day, divided into two doses of 20 mg each.

It has a "black box" warning for the possibility of severe rash. Common side effects can include sleepiness, drooling, constipation, or aggression. It is in the benzodiazepine class, but tends to produce less drowsiness and sleepiness than other medications in this group.

It is metabolized by the liver and can have some drug interactions, including reducing birth control effectiveness. It can have severe side effects and interactions with alcohol.

It is important to not stop this medication abruptly, as withdrawal seizures might occur.

Clonazepam (Klonopin)

This is a long-acting medication in the group called benzodiazepines. It is usually dosed twice per day. It may be used to treat seizures of several types, usually as an add-on (adjunctive) medication.

The most common side effect is drowsiness. Over time, the effectiveness of the medication may be lost, and the body may become used to it (tolerance), requiring higher doses. It is important to not stop this medication abruptly, as withdrawal seizures might occur.

Diazepam (Valium); rectal diazepam (Diastat)

This is also a medication in the benzodiazepine group. It is not often used as a regular AED, but more often as a "rescue medication"—something that can be dosed to provide short-term protection against seizures. When given by rectal route, it is absorbed rapidly and provides rapid short-term protection against further seizures. Like many benzodiazepines, the most common side effect is sleepiness or drowsiness. If taken regularly, it is important not to stop this medication abruptly, as withdrawal seizures might occur.

Eslicarbazepine (Aptiom)

This medication is approved for use in focal-onset seizures in people age 18 and older. It is quickly converted by the liver to the active form, which is later cleared by the kidneys.

A single dose lasts a long time (long "half-life") allowing it to be dosed just once per day. It is often started at 400 mg per day and gradually increased to a maximum of 1200 mg per day.

It is closely related to oxcarbazepine and has similar (although possibly fewer) side effects. Levels of this medication may be lower than expected if used with enzyme-inducing AEDs. It can also affect levels of other medications, including birth control pills.

Ethosuximide (Zarontin)

This medication is used for the treatment of absence seizures when they are not accompanied by other seizure types. It is not effective for treatment of generalized tonic-clonic seizures, and if someone has other seizure types along with absence seizures, an alternative medication, or another medication along with ethosuximide, must be used. It is mostly used in children with childhood absence epilepsy.

It is metabolized by the liver and has some potential medication interactions. Typical target blood levels are 40 mg/L to 100 mg/L. Dose-related side effects can include stomach upset, balance problems, and drowsiness. It can cause problems with blood counts and rash.

Ezogabine (Potiga)

This medication is approved as adjunctive (add-on) treatment for focal-onset seizures in people age 18 and older. It has a different mechanism (method of working) than other AEDs. It is believed to work by opening potassium channels on nerve cells (neurons).

It is dosed three times daily, starting at a low dose and gradually increasing as needed up to 400 mg three times daily.

Side effects can include urinary retention (difficulty urinating), which may require treatment. Dizziness and sleepiness can be seen. Side effects of changes in skin color and changes in the retina (back of the eye) have been reported. If this medication is used, it is important to be aware of these possible side effects, and periodic eye exams are required. It can interact with some other medications.

Felbamate (Felbatol)

Felbamate is not a first-line AED. This medication is approved for treatment of focal and secondarily generalized seizures in people over age 14 and the seizures of Lennox-Gastaut syndrome in children over age 2 *when the benefit is felt to outweigh the risk*. The prescribing information has prominent warnings about aplastic anemia (failure of the bone marrow to produce blood cells) and liver failure. Fatal cases of both have been attributed to felbamate use. A consent procedure should be followed if this medication is to be used. The purpose of the consent process is to ensure that the potential risks have been discussed and to document that the patient and doctor feel the risk is justified for the potential benefits.

It is usually dosed three times daily, beginning at low doses and increasing as needed to 3600 mg per day in divided doses. Careful monitoring of blood counts and liver function is required. In addition to the serious side effects mentioned, other side effects can include loss of appetite and weight loss, nausea, vomiting, difficulty sleeping, and headache. It can have multiple drug interactions with AEDs and other medications.

Gabapentin (Neurontin)

This medication is approved as adjunctive (add-on) treatment of focal and secondarily generalized tonic-clonic seizures in people over age 12 years and for the treatment of focal seizures in children between the ages of 3 and 12 years.

It does not undergo liver metabolism and is simply cleared by the kidneys. It does not have any important medication interactions. For treatment of seizures, it is dosed three times daily. After gradual start, the dose can be increased as needed to 1200 mg three times daily.

Dose-related side effects include dizziness, sleepiness, and balance problems. Longer-term use can cause weight gain and swelling of the legs and ankles.

Lacosamide (Vimpat)

Lacosamide is approved for use as adjunctive (add-on) therapy for the treatment of focal and secondarily generalized seizures in people age 17 or older. It is cleared by the kidneys and has no important drug interactions. It is dosed twice daily, beginning at low doses and increasing as needed to 200 mg twice daily.

Common dose-related side effects can include dizziness, nausea and vomiting, double or blurry vision, tremor, and balance problems.

Lamotrigine (Lamictal, Lamictal XR)

Lamotrigine is approved for the adjunctive (add-on) treatment of focal-onset and secondarily generalized seizures, for conversion to monotherapy (single drug) treatment, for the treatment of the seizures of Lennox-Gastaut syndrome in children over age 2, and for treatment of primary generalized tonic-clonic seizures in children over age 2 and adults. Standard lamotrigine is usually dosed twice daily; the extended-release form can be dosed once daily.

It has drug interactions with several AEDs, and use with these AEDs requires substantial changes in dosing. The levels of lamotrigine can also be affected by the use of hormonal contraception (birth control pills). Approximate blood level ranges are 2 to 10 mcg/mL for many people, although higher levels may be needed, if tolerated. Dose-related side effects can include headache, dizziness, balance problems, and either drowsiness or trouble sleeping (insomnia). It has warnings for severe rash, including Stevens-Johnson syndrome, and must be used with caution, especially in children.

Levetiracetam (Keppra, Keppra XR)

Levetiracetam is approved as adjunctive therapy for the treatment of focal-onset seizures in adults and children over age 4, for myoclonic seizures in juvenile myoclonic epilepsy for patients over age 12, and for adjunctive treatment of primary generalized epilepsy in adults and children over age 6. Standard levetiracetam is usually dosed twice daily; the extended-release form can be dosed once daily.

Levetiracetam is cleared by the kidneys without liver metabolism and has no known medication interactions. It is often started at 250 mg or 500 mg twice daily and can be gradually increased to 1500 mg twice daily if needed. The most common side effects are initial sleepiness and fatigue, and behavioral irritability.

Lorazepam (Ativan)

This is another medication in the benzodiazepine class. Like diazepam (Valium), it is rarely used as a routine AED but rather is often reserved for use as a "rescue medication"—for short-term use to provide intermittent seizure protection. The short-term protection provided is somewhat longer than that offered by diazepam. The main side effect is sleepiness. It can also be given intravenously (IV) by qualified medical personnel in emergency situations (for example, status epilepticus).

Oxcarbazepine (Trileptal, Oxtellar-XR)

Oxcarbazepine is approved as monotherapy or adjunctive (add-on) therapy for focal-onset seizures in adults, as monotherapy for children over age 4, and as adjunctive therapy for those over age 2 for treatment of focal-onset seizures. It is related to carbamazepine. Its properties make it somewhat easier to manage compared with carbamazepine, but it does still have known medication interactions, including with birth control pills and other antiepileptic medications. The standard form is usually dosed twice daily; the extended-release form can be given once daily.

Oxcarbazepine is often started at 300 mg twice daily and increased as needed up to a maximum of 2400 mg per day in divided doses. Dose-related side effects are similar to carbamazepine and can include dizziness, balance problems, double or blurry vision, drowsiness, and nausea. The possible side effect of low sodium levels in the blood is even more common than with carbamazepine. A rash can be seen as an allergic response, and those with a rash to carbamazepine are more likely to have a rash with oxcarbazepine treatment.

Perampanel (Fycompa)

Perampanel is approved for adjunctive (add-on) therapy for focal-onset seizures and primary generalized tonic-clonic seizures in people age 12 and older. It has a unique mechanism of action. It works by blocking excitation in the brain, specifically a type of glutamate (excitatory neurotransmitter) receptor. It has a long action in the body, which allows for once daily dosing. It is usually started at 2 mg per day and can be increased weekly up to 8 to 12 mg per day.

It has a "black box" (serious) warning for the possibility of serious psychiatric or behavioral reactions, including aggression and homicidal thinking. Common dose-related side effects can include dizziness, sleepiness, headaches, balance problems, weight gain, and irritability. It can interact with other AEDs and non-AEDs, including birth control pills.

Phenobarbital and Primidone

Phenobarbital has been in common use for more than 100 years but is used less today because of its relatively unfavorable side effect profile. It is used to treat focal and secondarily generalized seizures in adults and children. Primidone is a related medication that is broken down in the body to phenobarbital. Both medications have a long action in the body (long half-life), allowing once-daily dosing.

Both drugs are processed in the liver and are enzyme-inducing AEDs, and thus have multiple AED and non-AED drug interactions, including with birth control pills. Phenobarbital also comes in an intravenous (IV) form that is sometimes used by medical personnel to treat seizure emergencies (status epilepticus).

Common side effects are drowsiness, behavior problems, difficulty with learning, nausea, and unsteadiness. A rash as an allergic response can be seen, as well as decreases in blood counts. It can contribute to early osteoporosis.

Phenytoin (Dilantin, Fosphenytoin)

Phenytoin is used as monotherapy and adjunctive therapy for treatment of focal-onset seizures including secondarily generalized tonic-clonic seizures. Fosphenytoin is an intravenous (IV) form that is used as replacement therapy when someone is unable to take pills by mouth or in emergency situations (status epilepticus).

Its properties lead to many potential drug interactions with both AED and non-AED medications, including birth control pills. Its metabolism is unusual, making it sometimes difficult to maintain stable levels; small changes in dose can sometimes produce large changes in blood levels.

Common dose-related side effects include dizziness, balance problems, sleepiness, and incoordination. Rash, as part of an allergic response, can be seen, as well as rarely decreases in blood counts or liver problems. Long-term side effects can include coarsening of facial features, overgrowth of the gums, excess hair growth, peripheral neuropathy, bone loss/early osteoporosis, and atrophy (loss of size) of the cerebellum (part of the brain).

Pregabalin (Lyrica)

Pregabalin is approved for adjunctive (add-on) therapy for focal-onset seizures in adults. It is a close relative of and more potent version of gabapentin. It is cleared by the kidneys and not processed by the liver. It does not have known medication interactions. It is typically dosed twice daily for the treatment of seizures. It is often started at 50 to 100 mg per day and increased as needed to 300 mg twice daily.

Common side effects include drowsiness, weight gain, and ankle swelling.

Rufinamide (Banzel)

Rufinamide is approved for adjunctive treatment of Lennox-Gastaut syndrome in adults and children over age 4 years. In adults, it is dosed twice daily, starting at 200 to 400 mg and increasing gradually as needed up to a maximum of 3200 mg per day in divided doses.

Common dose-related side effects include dizziness, nausea and vomiting, tiredness, and double or blurred vision. Rarely can it cause problems with the liver or multiple organ systems. It has several potential interactions with other AEDs.

Sodium valproate (Depakote, Depakote ER; Depacon (intravenous form); Depakene (valproic acid—alternative form less often used)

Sodium valproate is used to treat both focal-onset and generalized seizure types. Several features of the drug make it prone to multiple medication interactions. The standard form is dosed two or three times per day; the extended-release form can often be given once daily. The intravenous form can be used when someone is unable to take medications by mouth (for example, following surgery) or in seizure emergencies (status epilepticus).

Common side effects can include tremor, stomach upset, diarrhea/loose stools, sleepiness, and unsteadiness. Low platelets (blood component that helps with clotting) can be seen; easy bruising or bleeding should be reported if it occurs. Serious side effects include liver problems (more common in young children) and pancreatitis (inflammation of the pancreas). Long-term effects can include higher risk of polycystic ovarian syndrome in women, hair loss, weight gain, and elevated ammonia in the blood. This medication is considered particularly high risk for causing birth defects.

Tiagabine (Gabitril)

Tiagabine is approved for adjunctive (add-on) treatment of focal-onset seizures in adults and children over age 12. It can potentially worsen seizures in people with generalized-from-onset seizures. It works by prolonging the action of GABA—the main inhibitory neurotransmitter in the brain. It is usually started at 4 mg per day and slowly increased as needed to up to 56 mg per day, divided at least twice daily, sometimes given three or four times daily.

Tiagabine may have interactions with other AEDs and non-AEDs. Common side effects can include tiredness, dizziness, decreased concentration, weakness, and depression.

Topiramate (Topamax, Trokendi-XR, Qudexy-XR)

Topiramate is approved as monotherapy and adjunctive therapy for focal-onset seizures in adults and children over age 2 years, as monotherapy or adjunctive therapy for primary generalized tonic-clonic seizures, and as adjunctive therapy for Lennox-Gastaut syndrome. It is usually started slowly at a low dose to help avoid problems with side effects. The standard form is usually given twice daily; the extended-release forms can be dosed once daily.

Topiramate can have drug interactions with AEDs and non-AEDs, including birth control pills. Common dose-related side effects can include dizziness, problems with concentration, and trouble with cognition, especially verbal skills. Less common but potentially serious side effects include a sudden onset of painful eye problems (acute angle-closure glaucoma). There is an increased risk of kidney stones. Topiramate may reduce the ability to sweat, leading to risk of heat stroke; this risk is higher in children. A rash may be seen as part of an allergic response. People with a history of allergies to sulfa drugs have an increased risk of rash on topiramate.

Vigabatrin (Sabril)

Vigabatrin is not a first-line AED because it can cause permanent, irreversible visual problems. Vigabatrin is approved as adjunctive therapy for focal-onset seizures in adults and for infantile spasms in children. Its use is restricted because of the risk of progressive visual field loss. Patients may not be aware of the visual loss until it is advanced. For this reason, the use of vigabatrin is restricted, and it is only prescribed through the SHARE program (http://sabril. net/hcp/prescribing_sabril/), which mandates discussion of risks and benefits of treatment and regular visual assessments during treatment.

Zonisamide (Zonegran)

Zonisamide is approved for use as adjunctive (add-on) treatment for focal-onset seizures in people over age 16. It is usually dosed twice daily, but its long action in the body (long half-life) permits once-daily dosing in some cases. It is usually started at a dose of 100 mg per day and increased as needed at two-week intervals to a maximum of 600 mg per day.

Dose-related side effects can include sleepiness, thinking (cognitive) problems, nausea, and dizziness. Less common but potentially serious side effects include kidney stones, decreased sweating/risk of heat stroke, and rash. People with a history of allergies to sulfa drugs may also have a rash with zonisamide. There is some potential for drug-drug interactions, including with other AEDs.

About the American Academy of Neurology

The American Academy of Neurology, an association of more than 30,000 neurologists and neuroscience professionals, is dedicated to promoting the highest quality patient-centered neurologic care. A neurologist is a doctor with specialized training in diagnosing, treating, and managing disorders of the brain and nervous system such as Alzheimer's disease, stroke, migraine, multiple sclerosis, concussion, Parkinson's disease, and epilepsy.

For more information about the American Academy of Neurology, visit *AAN.com*.

To sign up for a free subscription to *Neurology Now®*, the Academy's magazine for patients and caregivers, visit *NeurologyNow.com*.

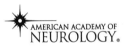

About the American Brain Foundation

The American Brain Foundation, the foundation of the American Academy of Neurology, supports crucial research and education to discover causes, improved treatments, and cures for the brain and other nervous system diseases. One in six people is affected by brain diseases such as Alzheimer's disease, traumatic brain injury, stroke, Parkinson's disease, multiple sclerosis, autism, and epilepsy.

For more information about the American Brain Foundation and how you can support research, visit *AmericanBrainFoundation.org*.

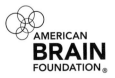

INDEX

References to figures, tables and boxes are denoted by an italicized *f*, *t*, and *b*.